My Keto Chaffle Cookbook

Fun and quick recipes to make before starting the day

Michelle Sells

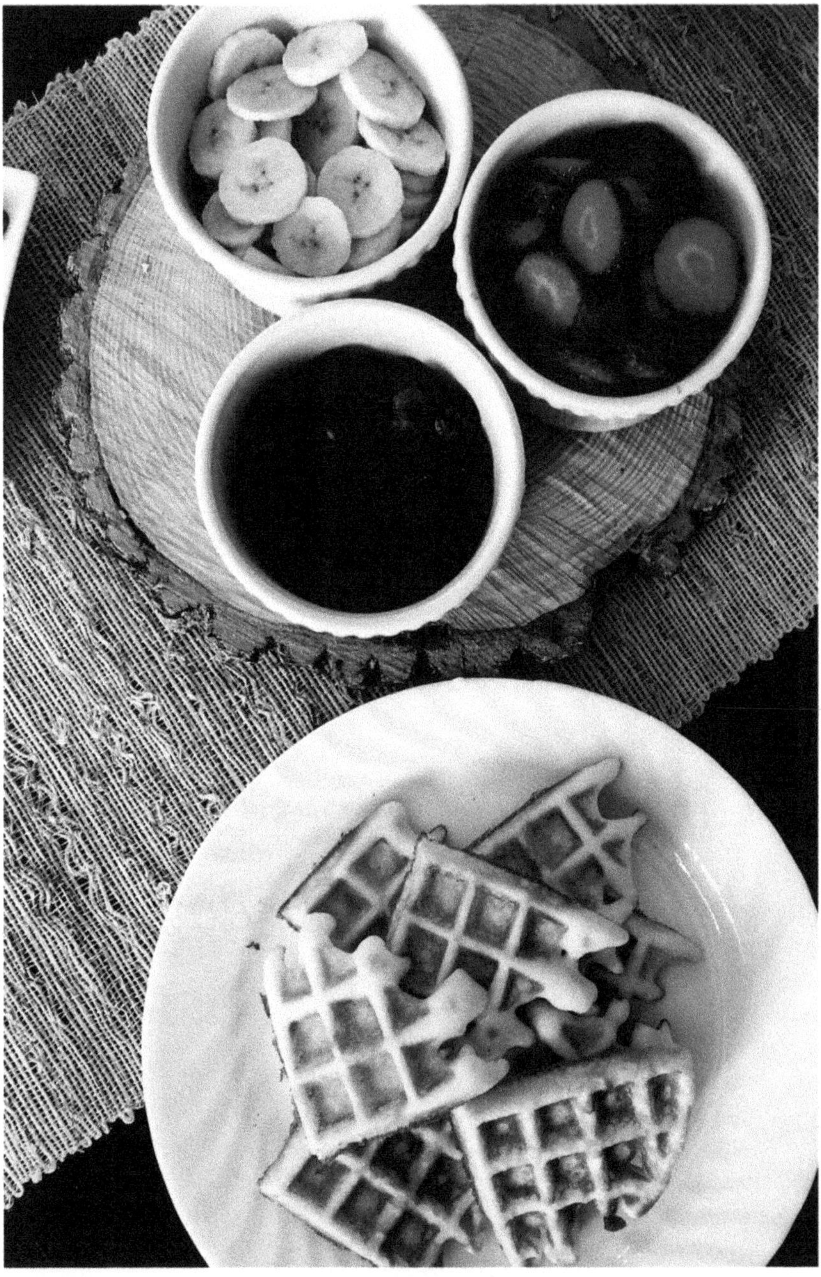

The content within this book has been derived from various sources. Please consult a licensed professional before attempting any techniques outlined in this book.

By reading this document, the reader agrees that under no circumstances is the author responsible for any losses, direct or indirect, which are incurred as a result of the use of information contained within this document, including, but not limited to, — errors, omissions, or inaccuracies.

Table of Contents

1 Mini Breakfast Chaffles

Servings:3

Cooking Time: 15 Minutes

Ingredients:

- 6 tsp coconut flour
- 1 tsp stevia
- 1/4 tsp baking powder
- 2 eggs
- 3 oz. cream cheese
- 1/2. tsp vanilla extract
- Topping
- 1 egg
- 6 slice bacon
- 2 oz. Raspberries for topping
- 2 oz. Blueberries for topping
- 2 oz. Strawberries for topping

Directions:

1. Heat up your square waffle maker and grease with cooking spray.
2. Mix together coconut flour, stevia, egg, baking powder, cheese and vanilla in mixing bowl.
3. Pour ½ of chaffles mixture in a waffle maker.
4. Close the lid and cook the chaffles for about 3-5 minutesutes.
5. Meanwhile, fry bacon slices in pan on medium heat for about 2-3 minutesutes until cooked and transfer themto plate.
6. In the same pan, fry eggs one by one in the leftover grease of bacon.
7. Once chaffles are cooked, carefully transferthem toplate.
8. Serve with fried eggs and bacon slice and berries on top.
9. Enjoy!

Nutrition Info:

PerServings: Protein: 16% 75 kcal Fat: 75% 346 kcal Carbohydrates: 9% 41 kcal

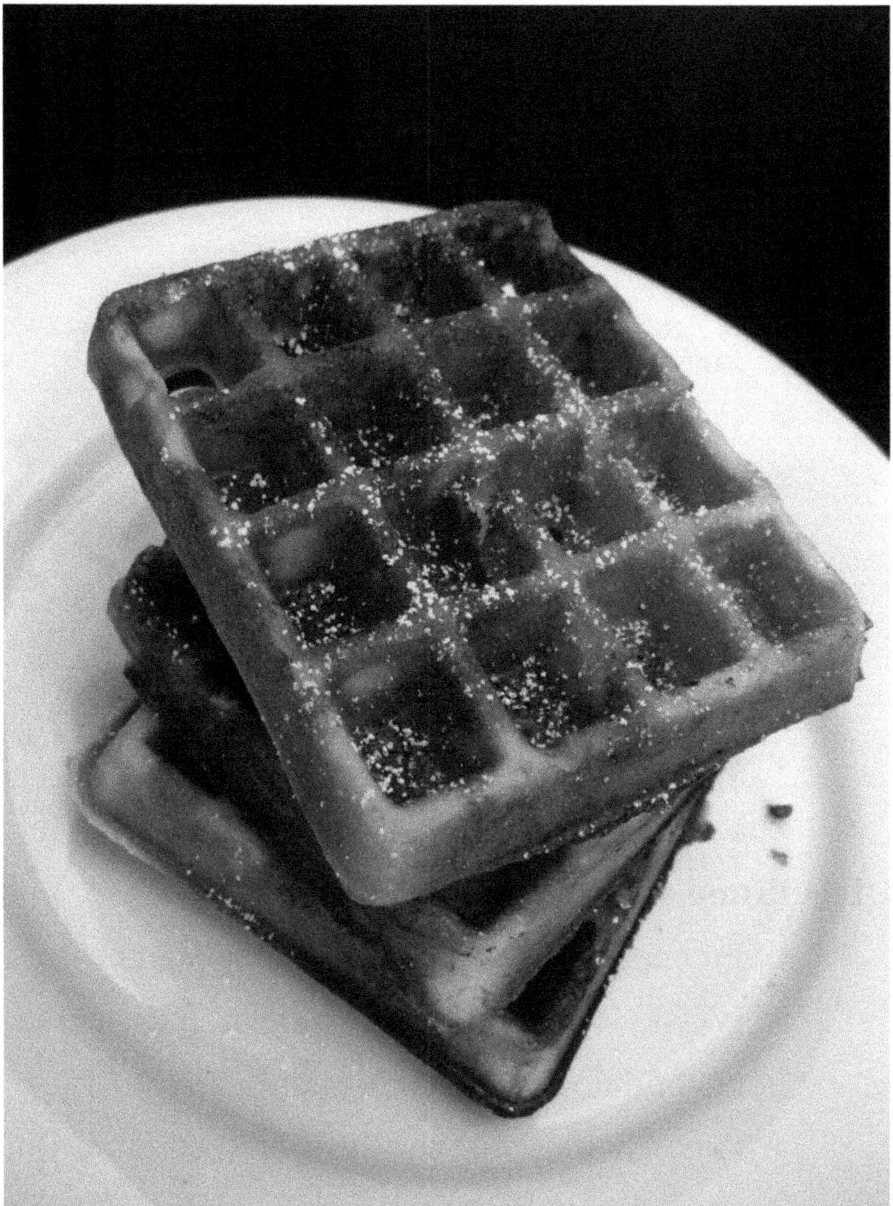

2 Crispy Chaffles With Egg & Asparagus

Servings:1

Cooking Time: 10 Minutes

Ingredients:

- 1 egg
- 1/4 cup cheddar cheese
- 2 tbsps. almond flour
- ½ tsp. baking powder
- TOPPING
- 1 egg
- 4-5 stalks asparagus
- 1 tsp avocado oil

Directions:

1. Preheat waffle maker to medium-high heat.
2. Whisk together egg, mozzarella cheese, almond flour, and baking powder
3. Pour chaffles mixture into the center of the waffle iron. Close the waffle maker and let cook for 5 minutesutes or until waffle is golden brown and set.

4. Remove chaffles from the waffle maker and serve.
5. Meanwhile, heat oil in a nonstick pan.
6. Once the pan is hot, fry asparagus for about 4-5 minutesutes until golden brown.
7. Poach the egg in boil water for about 2-3 minutesutes.
8. Once chaffles are cooked, remove from the maker.
9. Serve chaffles with the poached egg and asparagus.

Nutrition Info:

*perServings***:** Protein: 26% 85 kcal Fat: 69% 226 kcal Carbohydrates: 5% 16 kcal

3 Delicious Raspberriestaco Chaffles

Servings:1

Cooking Time: 15 Minutes

Ingredients:

- 1 egg white
- 1/4 cup jack cheese, shredded
- 1/4 cup cheddar cheese, shredded
- 1 tsp coconut flour
- 1/4 tsp baking powder
- 1/2 tsp stevia
- For Topping
- 4 oz. raspberries
- 2 tbsps. coconut flour
- 2 oz. unsweetened raspberry sauce

Directions:

1. Switch on yourround Waffle Maker and grease it with cooking spray once it is hot.
2. Mix together all chaffle ingredients in a bowl and combine with a fork.

3. Pour chaffle batter in a preheated maker and close the lid.
4. Roll the taco chaffle around using a kitchen roller, set it aside and allow it to set for a few minutesutes.
5. Once the taco chaffle is set, remove from the roller.
6. Dip raspberries in sauce and arrange on taco chaffle.
7. Drizzle coconut flour on top.
8. Enjoy raspberries taco chaffle with keto coffee.

Nutrition Info:

perServings: Protein: 28% 77 kcal Fat: 6 187 kcal Carbohydrates: 3% 8 kcal

4 Coconut Chaffles

Servings:2

Cooking Time: 5 Minutes

Ingredients:

- 1 egg
- 1 oz. cream cheese,
- 1 oz. cheddar cheese
- 2 tbsps. coconut flour
- 1 tsp. stevia
- 1 tbsp. coconut oil, melted
- 1/2 tsp. coconut extract
- 2 eggs, soft boil for serving

Directions:

1. Heat you minutesi Dash waffle maker and grease with cooking spray.
2. Mix together all chaffles ingredients in a bowl.
3. Pour chaffle batter in a preheated waffle maker.
4. Close the lid.

5. Cook chaffles for about 2-3 minutesutes until golden brown.
6. Serve with boil egg and enjoy!

Nutrition Info:

perServings: Protein: 21% 32 kcal Fat: % 117 kcal Carbohydrates: 3% 4 kcal

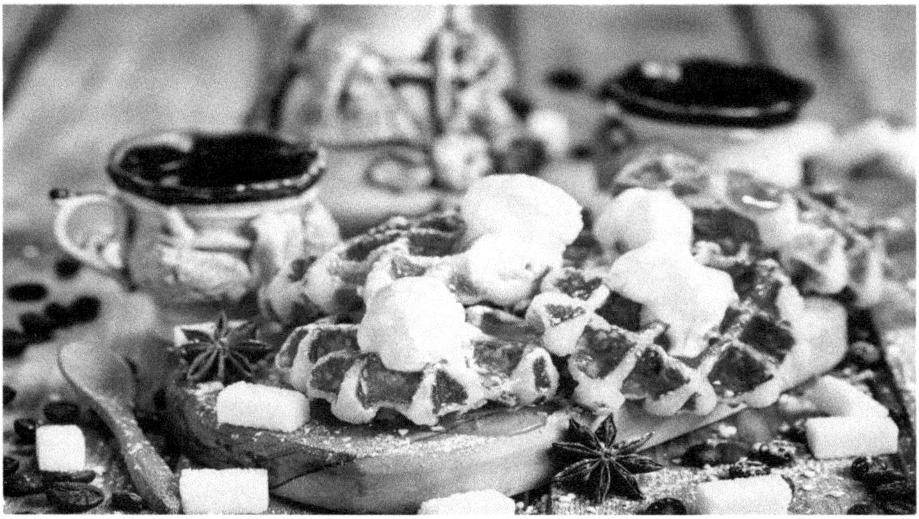

5 Garlic And Parsley Chaffles

Servings:1

Cooking Time: 5 Minutes

Ingredients:

- 1 large egg
- 1/4 cup cheese mozzarella
- 1 tsp. coconut flour
- ¼ tsp. baking powder
- ½ tsp. garlic powder
- 1 tbsp. minutesced parsley
- For Serving
- 1 Poach egg
- 4 oz. smoked salmon

Directions:

1. Switch on yourDash minutesiwaffle maker and let it preheat.
2. Grease waffle maker with cooking spray.

3. Mix together egg, mozzarella, coconut flour, baking powder, and garlic powder, parsley to a mixing bowl until combined well.
4. Pour batter in circle chaffle maker.
5. Close the lid.
6. Cook for about 2-3 minutesutes or until the chaffles are cooked.
7. Serve with smoked salmon and poached egg.
8. Enjoy!

Nutrition Info:

perServings: Protein: 45% 140 kcal Fat: 51% 160 kcal Carbohydrates: 4% 14 kcal

6 Scrambled Eggs On A Spring Onion

Chaffle

Servings:4

Cooking Time:7–9 Minutes

Ingredients:

- Batter
- 4 eggs
- 2 cups grated mozzarella cheese
- 2 spring onions, finely chopped
- Salt and pepper to taste
- ½ teaspoon dried garlic powder
- 2 tablespoons almond flour
- 2 tablespoons coconut flour
- Other
- 2 tablespoons butter for brushing the waffle maker
- 6-8 eggs
- Salt and pepper
- 1 teaspoon Italian spice mix
- 1 tablespoon olive oil

- 1 tablespoon freshly chopped parsley

Directions:

1. Preheat the waffle maker.
2. Crack the eggs into a bowl and add the grated cheese.
3. Mix until just combined, then add the chopped spring onions and season with salt and pepper and dried garlic powder.
4. Stir in the almond flour and mix until everything is combined.
5. Brush the heated waffle maker with butter and add a few tablespoons of the batter.
6. Close the lid and cook for about 7–8 minutes depending on your waffle maker.
7. While the chaffles are cooking, prepare the scrambled eggs by whisking the eggs in a bowl until frothy, about 2 minutes. Season with salt and black pepper to taste and add the Italian spice mix. Whisk to blend in the spices.
8. Warm the oil in a non-stick pan over medium heat.

9. Pour the eggs in the pan and cook until eggs are set to your liking.
10. Serve each chaffle and top with some scrambled eggs. Top with freshly chopped parsley.

Nutrition Info:

perServings: Calories 194, fat 14.7 g, carbs 5 g, sugar 0.6 g, Protein 1 g, sodium 191 mg

7 Egg On A Cheddar Cheese Chaffle

Servings:4

Cooking Time:7–9 Minutes

Ingredients:

- Batter
- 4 eggs
- 2 cups shredded white cheddar cheese
- Salt and pepper to taste
- Other
- 2 tablespoons butter for brushing the waffle maker
- 4 large eggs
- 2 tablespoons olive oil

Directions:

1. Preheat the waffle maker.
2. Crack the eggs into a bowl and whisk them with a fork.
3. Stir in the grated cheddar cheese and season with salt and pepper.

4. Brush the heated waffle maker with butter and add a few tablespoons of the batter.
5. Close the lid and cook for about 7–8 minutes depending on your waffle maker.
6. While chaffles are cooking, cook the eggs.
7. Warm the oil in a large non-stick pan that has a lid over medium-low heat for 2-3 minutes
8. Crack an egg in a small ramekin and gently add it to the pan. Repeat the same way for the other 3 eggs.
9. Cover and let cook for 2 to 2 ½ minutes for set eggs but with runny yolks.
10. Remove from heat.
11. To serve, place a chaffle on each plate and top with an egg. Season with salt and black pepper to taste.

Nutrition Info:

perServings: Calories 4 fat 34 g, carbs 2 g, sugar 0.6 g, Protein 26 g, sodium 518 mg

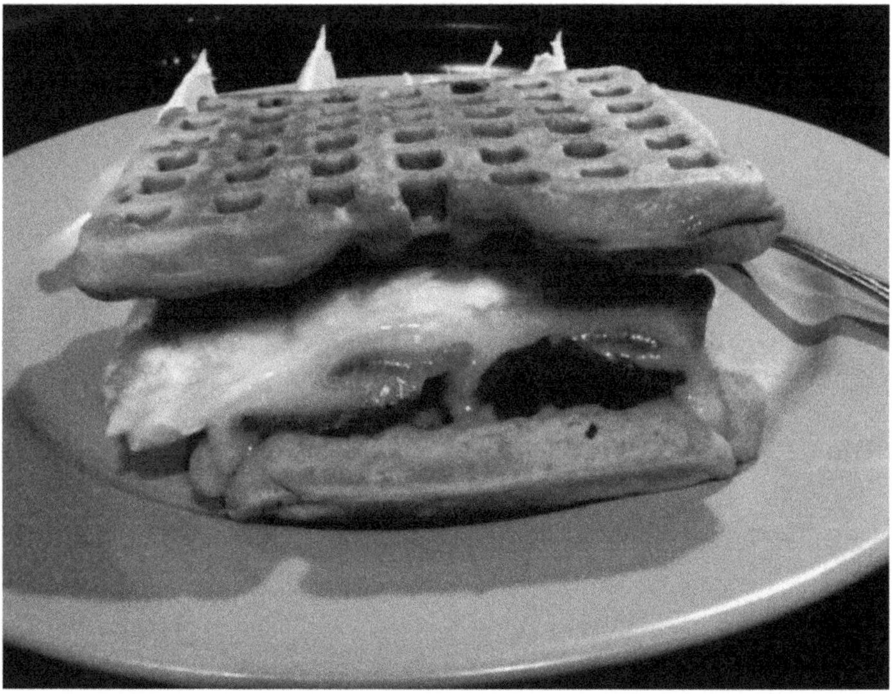

8 Avocado Chaffle Toast

Servings:3

Cooking Time: 10 Minutes

Ingredients:

- 4 tbsps. avocado mash
- 1/2 tsp lemon juice
- 1/8 tsp salt
- 1/8 tsp black pepper
- 2 eggs
- 1/2 cup shredded cheese
- For serving
- 3 eggs
- ½ avocado thinly sliced
- 1 tomato, sliced

Directions:

1. Mash avocado mash with lemon juice, salt, and black pepper in mixing bowl, until well combined.

2. In a small bowl beat egg and pour eggs in avocado mixture and mix well.
3. Switch on Waffle Maker to pre-heat.
4. Pour 1/8 of shredded cheese in a waffle maker and then pour ½ of egg and avocado mixture and then 1/8 shredded cheese.
5. Close the lid and cook chaffles for about 3 - 4 minutesutes.
6. Repeat with the remaining mixture.
7. Meanwhile,fry eggs in a pan for about 1-2 minutesutes.
8. For serving, arrange fried egg on chaffle toast with avocado slice and tomatoes.
9. Sprinkle salt and pepper on top and enjoy!

Nutrition Info:

perServings: Protein: 26% 66 kcal Fat: 67% 169 kcal Carbohydrates: 6% 15 kcal

9 Cajun & Feeta Chaffles

Servings:1

Cooking Time: 10 Minutes

Ingredients:

- 1 egg white
- 1/4 cup shredded mozzarella cheese
- 2 tbsps. almond flour
- 1 tsp Cajun Seasoning
- FOR SERVING
- 1 egg
- 4 oz. feta cheese
- 1 tomato, sliced

Directions:

1. Whisk together egg, cheese, and seasoning in a bowl.
2. Switch on and grease waffle maker with cooking spray.
3. Pour batter in a preheated waffle maker.
4. Cook chaffles for about 2-3 minutesutes until the chaffle is cooked through.

5. Meanwhile, fry the egg in a non-stick pan for about 1-2 minutesutes.
6. For serving set fried egg on chaffles with feta cheese and tomatoes slice.

Nutrition Info:

perServings*:* Protein: 28% 119 kcal Fat: 64% 2 kcal Carbohydrates: 7% 31 kcal

10 Crispy Chaffles With Sausage

Servings:2

Cooking Time: 10 Minutes

Ingredients:

- 1/2 cup cheddar cheese
- 1/2 tsp. baking powder
- 1/4 cup egg whites
- 2 tsp. pumpkin spice
- 1 egg, whole
- 2 chicken sausage
- 2 slice bacon
- salt and pepper to taste
- 1 tsp. avocado oil

Directions:

1. Mix together all ingredients in a bowl.
2. Allow batter to sit while waffle iron warms.
3. Spray waffle iron with nonstick spray.

4. Pour batter in the waffle maker and cook according to the directions of the manufacturer.
5. Meanwhile, heat oil in a pan and fry the egg, according to your choice and transfer it toa plate.
6. In the same pan, fry bacon slice and sausage on medium heat for about 2-3 minutesutes until cooked.
7. Once chaffles are cooked thoroughly, remove them from the maker.
8. Serve with fried egg, bacon slice, sausages and enjoy!

Nutrition Info:

perServings: Protein: 22% 86 kcal Fat: 74% 286 kcal Carbohydrates: 3% 12 kcal

11 Chili Chaffle

Servings:4

Cooking Time:7–9 Minutes

Ingredients:

- Batter
- 4 eggs
- ½ cup grated parmesan cheese
- 1½ cups grated yellow cheddar cheese
- 1 hot red chili pepper
- Salt and pepper to taste
- ½ teaspoon dried garlic powder
- 1 teaspoon dried basil
- 2 tablespoons almond flour
- Other
- 2 tablespoons olive oil for brushing the waffle maker

Directions:

1. Preheat the waffle maker.

2. Crack the eggs into a bowl and add the grated parmesan and cheddar cheese.
3. Mix until just combined and add the chopped chili pepper. Season with salt and pepper, dried garlic powder and dried basil. Stir in the almond flour.
4. Mix until everything is combined.
5. Brush the heated waffle maker with olive oil and add a few tablespoons of the batter.
6. Close the lid and cook for about 7–8 minutes depending on your waffle maker.

Nutrition Info:

perServings: Calories 36 fat 30.4 g, carbs 3.1 g, sugar 0.7 g, Protein 21.5 g, sodium 469 mg

12 Simple Savory Chaffle

Servings:4

Cooking Time: 7–9 Minutes

Ingredients:

- Batter
- 4 eggs
- 1 cup grated mozzarella cheese
- 1 cup grated provolone cheese
- ½ cup almond flour
- 2 tablespoons coconut flour
- 2½ teaspoons baking powder
- Salt and pepper to taste
- Other
- 2 tablespoons butter to brush the waffle maker

Directions:

1. Preheat the waffle maker.
2. Add the grated mozzarella and provolone cheese to a bowl and mix.

3. Add the almond and coconut flour and baking powder and season with salt and pepper.
4. Mix with a wire whisk and crack in the eggs.
5. Stir everything together until batter forms.
6. Brush the heated waffle maker with butter and add a few tablespoons of the batter.
7. Close the lid and cook for about 8 minutes depending on your waffle maker.
8. Serve and enjoy.

Nutrition Info:

perServings: Calories 352, fat 27.2 g, carbs 8.3 g, sugar 0.5 g, Protein 15 g, sodium 442 mg

13 Pizza Chaffle

Servings:4

Cooking Time:7–9 Minutes

Ingredients:

- Batter
- 4 eggs
- 1½ cups grated mozzarella cheese
- ½ cup grated parmesan cheese
- 2 tablespoons tomato sauce
- ¼ cup almond flour
- 1½ teaspoons baking powder
- Salt and pepper to taste
- 1 teaspoon dried oregano
- ¼ cup sliced salami
- Other
- 2 tablespoons olive oil for brushing the waffle maker
- ¼ cup tomato sauce for serving

Directions:

1. Preheat the waffle maker.
2. Add the grated mozzarella and grated parmesan to a bowl and mix.
3. Add the almond flour and baking powder and season with salt and pepper and dried oregano.
4. Mix with a wooden spoon or wire whisk and crack in the eggs.
5. Stir everything together until batter forms.
6. Stir in the chopped salami.
7. Brush the heated waffle maker with olive oil and add a few tablespoons of the batter.
8. Close the lid and cook for about 7–minutes depending on your waffle maker.
9. Serve with extra tomato sauce on top and enjoy.

Nutrition Info:

perServings: Calories 319, fat 25.2 g, carbs 5.9 g, sugar 1.7 g, Protein 19.3 g, sodium 596 mg

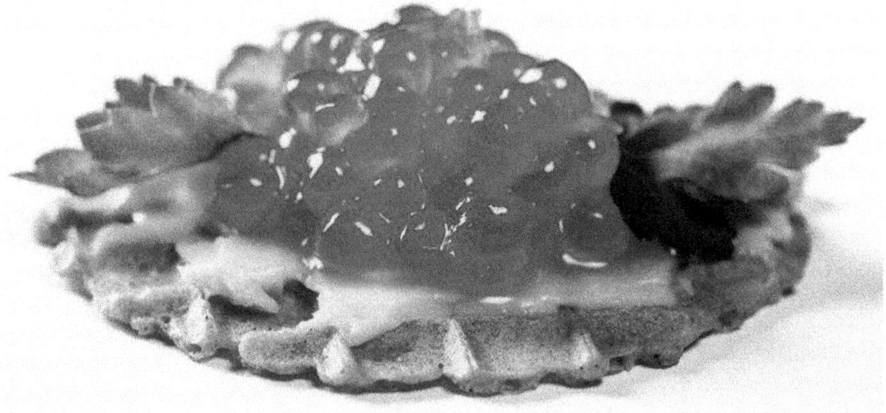

14 Bacon Chaffle

Servings:4

Cooking Time:7–9 Minutes

Ingredients:

- Batter
- 4 eggs
- 2 cups shredded mozzarella
- 2 ounces finely chopped bacon
- Salt and pepper to taste
- 1 teaspoon dried oregano
- Other
- 2 tablespoons olive oil for brushing the waffle maker

Directions:

1. Preheat the waffle maker.
2. Crack the eggs into a bowl and add the grated mozzarella cheese.
3. Mix until just combined and stir in the chopped bacon.

4. Season with salt and pepper and dried oregano.
5. Brush the heated waffle maker with olive oil and add a few tablespoons of the batter.
6. Close the lid and cook for about 7–8 minutes depending on your waffle maker.

Nutrition Info:

perServings: Calories 241, fat 19.8 g, carbs 1.3 g, sugar 0.4 g, Protein 14.8 g, sodium 4 mg

15 Chaffles Breakfast Bowl

Servings:2

Cooking Time: 5 Minutes

Ingredients:

- 1 egg
- 1/2 cup cheddar cheese shredded
- pinch of Italian seasoning
- 1 tbsp. pizza sauce
- TOPPING
- 1/2 avocado sliced
- 2 eggs boiled
- 1 tomato, halves
- 4 oz. fresh spinach leaves

Directions:

1. Preheat yourwaffle maker and grease with cooking spray.
2. Crack an egg in a small bowl and beat with Italian seasoning and pizza sauce.

3. Add shredded cheese to the egg and spices mixture.
4. Pour 1 tbsp. shredded cheese in a waffle maker and cook for 30 sec.
5. Pour Chaffles batter inthe waffle maker and close the lid.
6. Cook chaffles for about 4 minutesutes until crispy and brown.
7. Carefully remove chaffles from the maker.
8. Serve on the bed of spinach with boil egg, avocado slice, and tomatoes.
9. Enjoy!

Nutrition Info:

perServings: Protein: 23% 77 kcal Fat: 66% 222 kcal Carbohydrates: 11% 39 kcal

16 Morning Chaffles With Berries

Servings: 4

Cooking Time: 5 Minutes

Ingredients:

- 1 cup egg whites
- 1 cup cheddar cheese, shredded
- ¼ cup almond flour
- ¼ cup heavy cream
- TOPPING
- 4 oz. raspberries
- 4 oz. strawberries.
- 1 oz. keto chocolate flakes
- 1 oz. feta cheese.

Directions:

1. Preheat your square waffle maker and grease with cooking spray.
2. Beat egg white in a small bowl with flour.
3. Add shredded cheese to the egg whites and flour mixture and mix well.

4. Add cream and cheese tothe egg mixture.
5. Pour Chaffles batter in a waffle maker and close the lid.
6. Cook chaffles for about 4 minutesutes until crispy and brown.
7. Carefully remove chaffles from the maker.
8. Serve with berries, cheese, and chocolate on top.
9. Enjoy!

Nutrition Info:

perServings: Protein: 28% 68 kcal Fat: 67% 163 kcal Carbohydrates: 5% 12 kcal

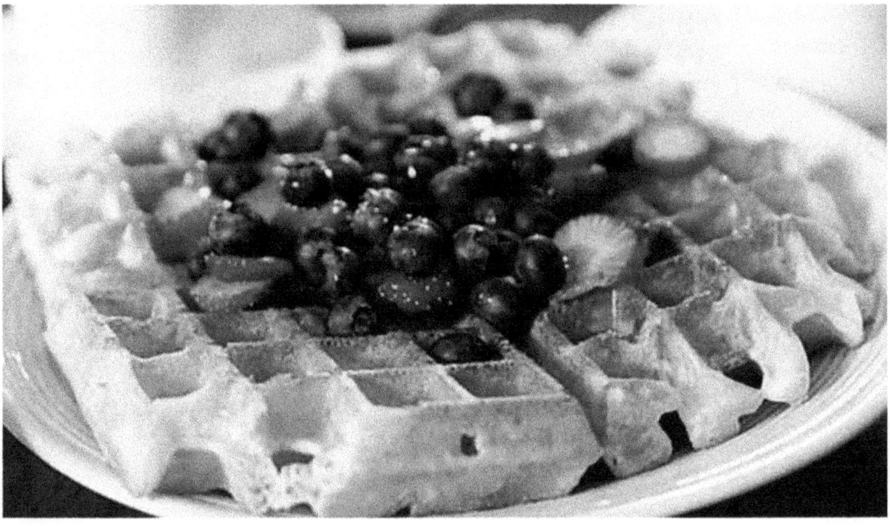

17 Chicken Bites With Chaffles

Servings: 2

Cooking Time: 10 minutes

Ingredients:

- 1 chicken breastscut into 2 x2 inch chunks
- 1 egg, whisked
- 1/4 cup almond flour
- 2 tbsps. onion powder
- 2 tbsps. garlic powder
- 1 tsp. dried oregano
- 1 tsp. paprika powder
- 1 tsp. salt
- 1/2 tsp. black pepper
- 2 tbsps. avocado oil

Directions:

1. Add all the dry ingredients together into a large bowl.Mix well.
2. Place the eggs into a separate bowl.

3. Dip each chicken piece into the egg and then into the dry ingredients.
4. Heat oil in 10-inch skillet, add oil.
5. Once avocado oil is hot, place the coated chicken nuggets onto a skillet and cook for 6-8 minutesutes until cooked and golden brown.
6. Serve with chaffles and raspberries.
7. Enjoy!

Nutrition Info:

perServings: Total Calories 401 kcal Fats 219 g Protein 32.35 g NetCarbs 1.46 g Fiber 3 g

18 Crunchy Fish And Chaffle Bites

Servings:4

Cooking Time: 15 Minutes

Ingredients:

- 1 lb. cod fillets, sliced into 4 slice
- 1 tsp. sea salt
- 1 tsp. garlic powder
- 1 egg, whisked
- 1 cup almond flour
- 2 tbsp. avocado oil
- CHAFFLE Ingredients:
- 2 eggs
- 1/2 cup cheddar cheese
- 2 tbsps. almond flour
- ½ tsp. Italian seasoning

Directions:

1. Mix together chaffle ingredients in a bowl and make 4 square
2. Put the chaffles in a preheated chaffle maker.

3. Mix together the salt, pepper, and garlic powder in a mixing bowl. Toss the cod cubes in this mixture and let sit for 10 minutesutes.
4. Then dip each cod slice into the egg mixture and then into the almond flour.
5. Heat oil in skillet and fish cubes for about 2-3 minutesutes, until cooked and browned
6. Serve on chaffles and enjoy!

Nutrition Info:

perServings*:* Protein: 38% 121 kcal Fat: 59% 189 kcal Carbohydrates: 3% 11 kcal

19 Grill Pork Chaffle Sandwich

Servings:2

Cooking Time: 15 Minutes

Ingredients:

- 1/2 cup mozzarella, shredded
- 1 egg
- I pinch garlic powder
- PORK PATTY
- 1/2 cup pork, minutesced
- 1 tbsp. green onion, diced
- 1/2 tsp Italian seasoning
- Lettuce leaves

Directions:

1. Preheat the square waffle maker and grease with
2. Mix together egg, cheese and garlic powder in a small mixing bowl.
3. Pour batter in a preheated waffle maker and close the lid.
4. Make 2 chaffles from thisbatter.

5. Cook chaffles for about 2-3 minutesutes until cooked through.
6. Meanwhile, mix together pork patty ingredients in a bowl and make 1 large patty.
7. Grill pork patty in a preheated grill for about 3-4 minutesutes per side until cooked through.
8. Arrange pork patty between two chaffles with lettuce leaves. Cut sandwich to make a triangular sandwich.
9. Enjoy!

Nutrition Info:

perServings*:* Protein: 48% 85 kcal Fat: 48% 86 kcal Carbohydrates: 4% 7 kcal

20 Chaffle & Chicken Lunch Plate

Servings:1

Cooking Time: 15 Minutes

Ingredients:

- 1 large egg
- 1/2 cup jack cheese, shredded
- 1 pinch salt
- For Serving
- 1 chicken leg
- salt
- pepper
- 1 tsp. garlic, minutesced
- 1 egg
- I tsp avocado oil

Directions:

1. Heat your square waffle maker and grease with cooking spray.
2. Pour Chaffle batter intothe skillet and cook for about 3 minutesutes.

3. Meanwhile,heat oil in a pan, over medium heat.
4. Once the oil is hot, add chicken thigh and garlicthen, cook for about 5 minutesutes. Flip and cook for another 3-4 minutesutes.
5. Season with salt and pepper and give them a good mix.
6. Transfer cooked thigh to plate.
7. Fry the egg in the same pan for about 1-2 minutesutes according to your choice.
8. Once chaffles are cooked, serve with fried egg and chicken thigh.
9. Enjoy!

Nutrition Info:

perServings: Protein: 31% 138 kcal Fat: 66% 292 kcal Carbohydrates: 2% kcal

21 Chaffle Egg Sandwich

Servings: 2

Cooking Time: 10 Minutes

Ingredients:

- 2 minutesI keto chaffle
- 2 slice cheddar cheese
- 1 egg simple omelet

Directions:

1. Prepare your oven on 4000 F.
2. Arrange egg omelet and cheese slice between chaffles.
3. Bake in the preheated oven for about 4-5 minutesutes until cheese is melted.
4. Once the cheese is melted, remove from the oven.
5. Serve and enjoy!

Nutrition Info:

perServings: Protein: 29% 144 kcal Fat: % 337 kcal Carbohydrates: 3% 14 kcal

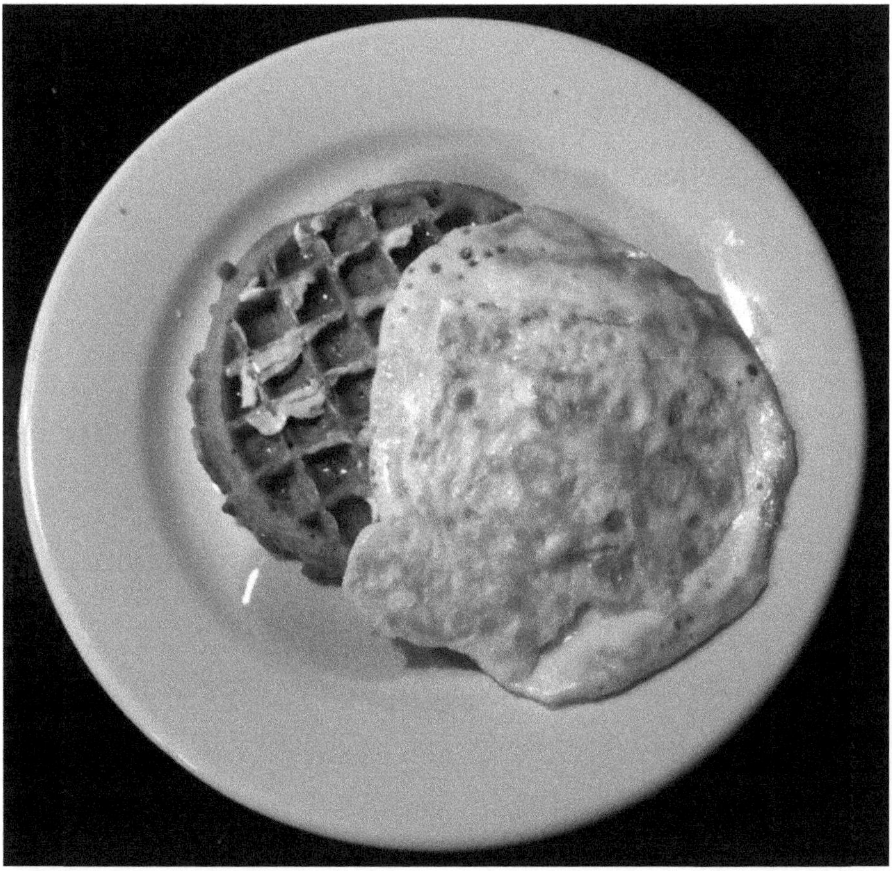

22 Chaffle Minutesi Sandwich

Servings: 2

Cooking Time: 10 Minutes

Ingredients:

- 1 large egg
- 1/8 cup almond flour
- 1/2 tsp. garlic powder
- 3/4 tsp. baking powder
- 1/2 cup shredded cheese
- SANDWICH FILLING
- 2 slices deli ham
- 2 slices tomatoes
- 1 slice cheddar cheese

Directions:

1. Grease your square waffle maker and preheat it on medium heat.
2. Mix together chaffle ingredients in a mixing bowl until well combined.

3. Pour batter intoa square waffle and make two chaffles.
4. Once chaffles are cooked, remove from the maker.
5. For a sandwich,arrange deli ham, tomato slice and cheddar cheese between two chaffles.
6. Cut sandwich from the center.
7. Serve and enjoy!

Nutrition Info:

perServings: Protein: 29% 70 kcal Fat: 66% 159 kcal Carbohydrates: 4% 10 kcal

23 Chaffle Cheese Sandwich

Servings: 1

Cooking Time: 10 Minutes

Ingredients:

- 2 square keto chaffle
- 2 slice cheddar cheese
- 2 lettuce leaves

Directions:

1. Prepare your oven on 4000 F.
2. Arrange lettuce leave and cheese slice between chaffles.
3. Bake in the preheated oven for about 4-5 minutesutes until cheese is melted.
4. Once the cheese is melted, remove from the oven.
5. Serve and enjoy!

Nutrition Info:

perServings: Protein: 28% kcal Fat: 69% 149 kcal Carbohydrates: 3% 6 kcal

24 Chicken Zinger Chaffle

Servings:2

Cooking Time: 15 Minutes

Ingredients:

- 1 chicken breast, cut into 2 pieces
- 1/2 cup coconut flour
- 1/4 cup finely grated Parmesan
- 1 tsp. paprika
- 1/2 tsp. garlic powder
- 1/2 tsp. onion powder
- 1 tsp. salt& pepper
- 1 egg beaten
- Avocado oil for frying
- Lettuce leaves
- BBQ sauce
- CHAFFLE Ingredients:
- 4 oz. cheese
- 2 whole eggs
- 2 oz. almond flour

- 1/4 cup almond flour
- 1 tsp baking powder

Directions:

1. Mix together chaffle ingredients in a bowl.
2. Pour the chaffle batter in preheated greased square chaffle maker.
3. Cook chaffles for about 2-minutesutes until cooked through.
4. Make square chaffles from this batter.
5. Meanwhile mix together coconut flour, parmesan, paprika, garlic powder, onion powder salt and pepper in a bowl.
6. Dip chicken first in coconut flour mixture then in beaten egg.
7. Heat avocado oil in a skillet and cook chicken from both sides. until lightly brown and cooked
8. Set chicken zinger between two chaffles with lettuce and BBQ sauce.
9. Enjoy!

Nutrition Info:

perServings: Protein: 30% 219 kcal Fat: 60% 435 kcal Carbohydrates: 9% 66 kcal

25 Double Chicken Chaffles

Servings:2

Cooking Time: 5 Minutes

Ingredients:

- 1/2 cup boil shredded chicken
- 1/4 cup cheddar cheese
- 1/8 cup parmesan cheese
- 1 egg
- 1 tsp. Italian seasoning
- 1/8 tsp. garlic powder
- 1 tsp. cream cheese

Directions:

1. Preheat the Belgian waffle maker.
2. Mix together in chaffle ingredients in a bowl and mix together.
3. Sprinkle 1 tbsp. of cheese in a waffle maker and pour in chaffle batter.
4. Pour 1 tbsp. of cheese over batter and close the lid.
5. Cook chaffles for about 4 to minutesutes.

6. Serve with a chicken zinger and enjoy the double chicken flavor.

Nutrition Info:

perServings: Protein: 30% 60 kcal Fat: 65% 129 kcal Carbohydrates: 5% 9 kcal

27 Chaffles With Topping

Servings: 3

Cooking Time: 10 Minutes

Ingredients:

- 1 large egg
- 1 tbsp. almond flour
- 1 tbsp. full-fat Greek yogurt
- 1/8 tsp baking powder
- 1/4 cup shredded Swiss cheese
- TOPPING
- 4oz. grillprawns
- 4 oz. steamed cauliflower mash
- 1/2 zucchini sliced
- 3 lettuce leaves
- 1 tomato, sliced
- 1 tbsp. flax seeds

Directions:

1. Make 3 chaffles with the given chaffles ingredients.

2. For serving, arrange lettuce leaves on each chaffle.
3. Top with zucchini slice, grill prawns, cauliflower mash and a tomato slice.
4. Drizzle flax seeds on top.
5. Serve and enjoy!

Nutrition Info:

perServings: Protein: 45% 71 kcal Fat: 47% 75 kcal Carbohydrates: 8% 12 kcal

28 Chaffle With Cheese & Bacon

Servings:2

Cooking Time: 15 Minutes

Ingredients:

- 1 egg
- 1/2 cup cheddar cheese, shredded
- 1 tbsp. parmesan cheese
- 3/4 tsp coconut flour
- 1/4 tsp baking powder
- 1/8 tsp Italian Seasoning
- pinch of salt
- 1/4 tsp garlic powder
- FOR TOPPING
- 1 bacon sliced, cooked and chopped
- 1/2 cup mozzarella cheese, shredded
- 1/4 tsp parsley, chopped

Directions:

1. Preheat oven to 400 degrees.
2. Switch on your minutesi waffle maker and grease with cooking spray.
3. Mix together chaffle ingredients in a mixing bowl until combined.
4. Spoon half of the batter in the center of the waffle maker and close the lid. Cook chaffles for about 3-minutesutes until cooked.
5. Carefully remove chaffles from the maker.
6. Arrange chaffles in a greased baking tray.
7. Top with mozzarella cheese, chopped bacon and parsley.
8. And bake in the oven for 4 -5 minutesutes.
9. Once the cheese is melted, remove from the oven.
10. Serve and enjoy!

Nutrition Info:

perServings: Protein: 28% 90 kcal Fat: 69% 222 kcal Carbohydrates: 3% kcal

29 Grill Beefsteak And Chaffle

Servings: 1

Cooking Time: 10 Minutes

Ingredients:

- 1 beefsteak rib eye
- 1 tsp salt
- 1 tsp pepper
- 1 tbsp. lime juice
- 1 tsp garlic

Directions:

1. Prepare your grill for direct heat.
2. Mix together all spices and rub over beefsteak evenly.
3. Place the beef on the grill rack over medium heat.
4. Cover and cook steak for about6 to 8 minutesutes. Flip and cook for another 5 minutesutes until cooked through.
5. Serve with keto simple chaffle and enjoy!

Nutrition Info:

perServings: Protein: 51% 274 kcal Fat: 45% 243 kcal Carbohydrates: 4% 22 kcal

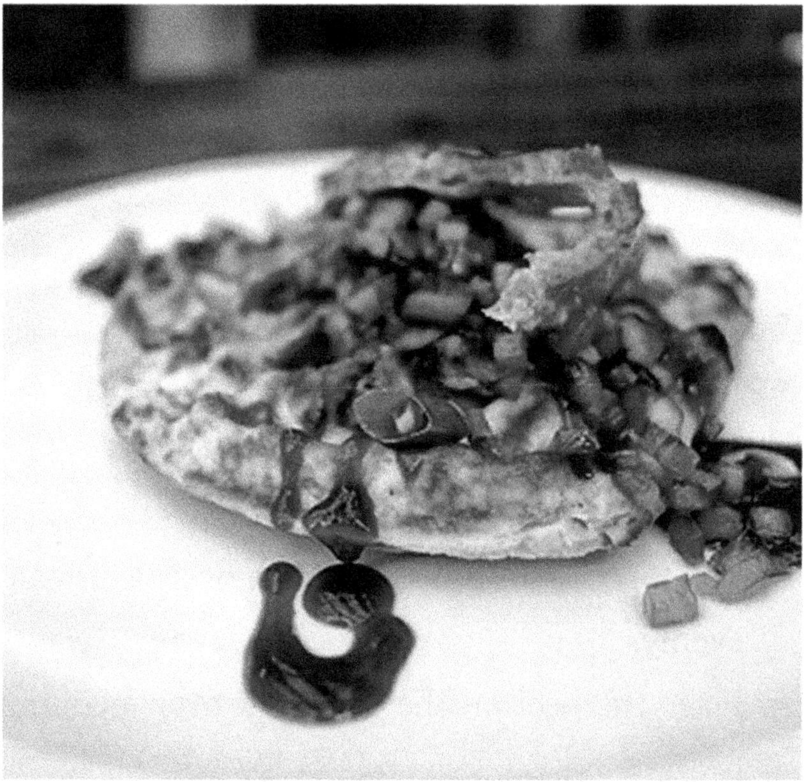

30 Cauliflower Chaffles And Tomatoes

Servings:2

Cooking Time: 15 Minutes

Ingredients:

- 1/2 cup cauliflower
- 1/4 tsp. garlic powder
- 1/4 tsp. black pepper
- 1/4 tsp. Salt
- 1/2 cup shredded cheddar cheese
- 1 egg
- FOR TOPPING
- 1 lettuce leave
- 1 tomato sliced
- 4 oz. cauliflower steamed, mashed
- 1 tsp sesame seeds

Directions:

1. Add all chaffle ingredients into a blender and mix well.

2. Sprinkle 1/8 shredded cheese on the waffle maker and pour cauliflower mixture in a preheated waffle maker and sprinkle the rest of the cheese over it.
3. Cook chaffles for about 4-5 minutesutes until cooked
4. For serving, lay lettuce leaves over chaffle top with steamed cauliflower and tomato.
5. Drizzle sesame seeds on top.
6. Enjoy!

Nutrition Info:

perServings: Protein: 25% 49 kcal Fat: 65% 128 kcal Carbohydrates: 10% 21 kcal

31 Layered Cheese Chaffles

Servings: 1

Cooking Time: 5 Minutes

Ingredients:

- 1 organic egg, beaten
- 1/3 cup Cheddar cheese, shredded
- ½ teaspoon ground flaxseed
- ¼ teaspoon organic baking powder
- 2 tablespoons Parmesan cheese, shredded

Directions:

1. Preheat a mini waffle iron and then grease it.
2. In a bowl, place all the ingredients except Parmesan and beat until well combined.
3. Place half the Parmesan cheese in the bottom of preheated waffle iron.
4. Place half of the egg mixture over cheese and top with the remaining Parmesan cheese.
5. Cook for about 3-minutes or until golden brown.
6. Serve warm.

Nutrition Info:

perServings: Calories: 264Net Carb: 1.Fat: 20gSaturated Fat: 11.1gCarbohydrates: 2.1gDietary Fiber: 0.4g Sugar: 0.6gProtein: 18.9g

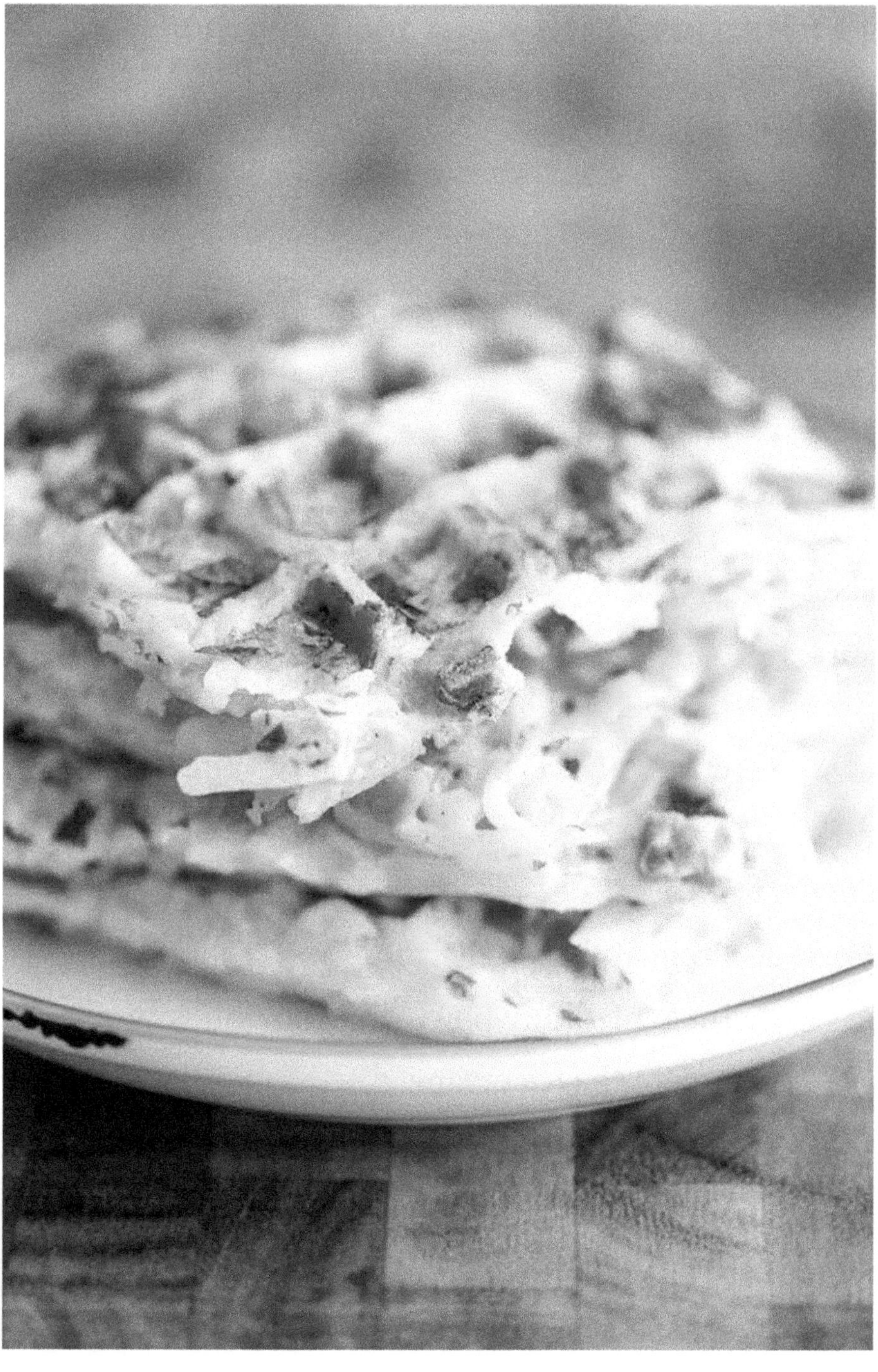

32 Chaffles With Keto Ice Cream

Servings: 2

Cooking Time: 14 Minutes

Ingredients:

- 1 egg, beaten
- ½ cup finely grated mozzarella cheese
- ¼ cup almond flour
- 2 tbsp swerve confectioner's sugar
- 1/8 tsp xanthan gum
- Low-carb ice cream (flavor of your choice) for serving

Directions:

1. Preheat the waffle iron.
2. In a medium bowl, mix all the ingredients except the ice cream.
3. Open the iron and add half of the mixture. Close and cook until crispy, 7 minutes.
4. Transfer the chaffle to a plate and make second one with the remaining batter.

5. On each chaffle, add a scoop of low carb ice cream, fold into half-moons and enjoy.

Nutrition Info:

perServings: Calories 89Fats 48gCarbs 1.67gNet Carbs 1.37gProtein 5.91g

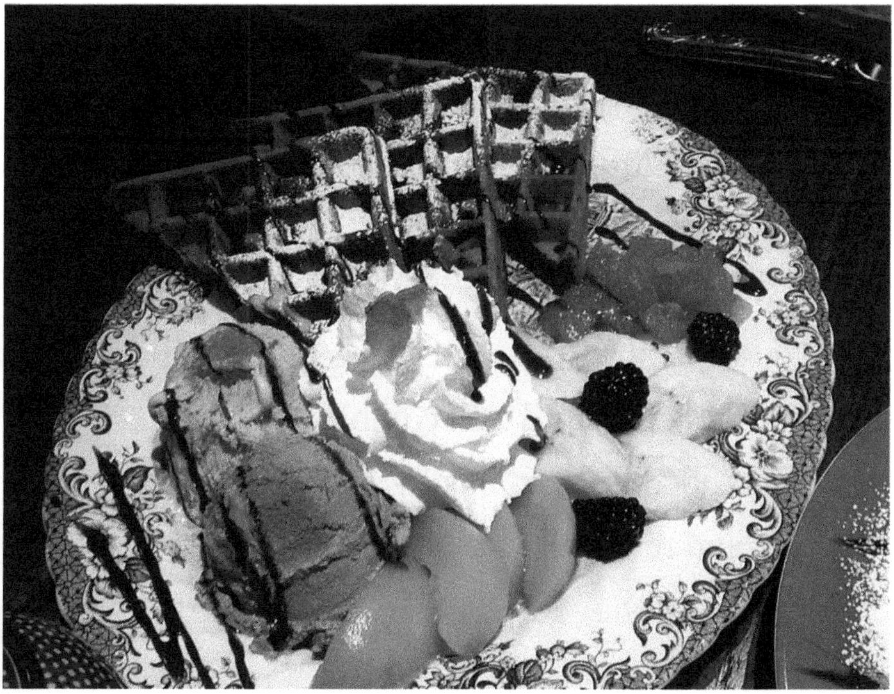

33 Vanilla Mozzarella Chaffles

Servings: 2

Cooking Time: 12 Minutes

Ingredients:

- 1 organic egg, beaten
- 1 teaspoon organic vanilla extract
- 1 tablespoon almond flour
- 1 teaspoon organic baking powder
- Pinch of ground cinnamon
- 1 cup Mozzarella cheese, shredded

Directions:

1. Preheat a mini waffle iron and then grease it.
2. In a bowl, place the egg and vanilla extract and beat until well combined.
3. Add the flour, baking powder and cinnamon and mix well.
4. Add the Mozzarella cheese and stir to combine.
5. In a small bowl, place the egg and Mozzarella cheese and stir to combine.

6. Place half of the mixture into preheated waffle iron and cook for about 5-minutes or until golden brown.
7. Repeat with the remaining mixture.
8. Serve warm.

Nutrition Info:

perServings: Calories: 103Net Carb: 2.4gFat: 6.6gSaturated Fat: 2.3gCarbohydrates: 2.Dietary Fiber: 0.5g Sugar: 0.6gProtein: 6.8g

34 Bruschetta Chaffle

Servings: 2

Cooking Time: 5 Minutes

Ingredients:

- 2 basic chaffles
- 2 tablespoons sugar-free marinara sauce
- 2 tablespoons mozzarella, shredded
- 1 tablespoon olives, sliced
- 1 tomato sliced
- 1 tablespoon keto friendly pesto sauce
- Basil leaves

Directions:

1. Spread marinara sauce on each chaffle.
2. Spoon pesto and spread on top of the marinara sauce.
3. Top with the tomato, olives and mozzarella.
4. Bake in the oven for 3 minutes or until the cheese has melted.
5. Garnish with basil.
6. Serve and enjoy.

Nutrition Info:

perServings: Calories 182Total Fat 11g Saturated Fat 6.1g Cholesterol 30mg Sodium 508mg Potassium 1mgTotal Carbohydrate 3.1g Dietary Fiber 1.1g Protein 16.8g Total Sugars 1g

35 Egg-free Psyllium Husk Chaffles

Servings: 1

Cooking Time: 4 Minutes

Ingredients:

- 1 ounce Mozzarella cheese, shredded
- 1 tablespoon cream cheese, softened
- 1 tablespoon psyllium husk powder

Directions:

1. Preheat a waffle iron and then grease it.
2. In a blender, place all ingredients and pulse until a slightly crumbly mixture forms.
3. Place the mixture into preheated waffle iron and cook for about 4 minutes or until golden brown.
4. Serve warm.

Nutrition Info:

perServings: Calories: 137Net Carb: 1.3gFat: 8.8gSaturated Fat: 2gCarbohydrates: 1.3gDietary Fiber: 0g Sugar: 0gProtein: 9.5g

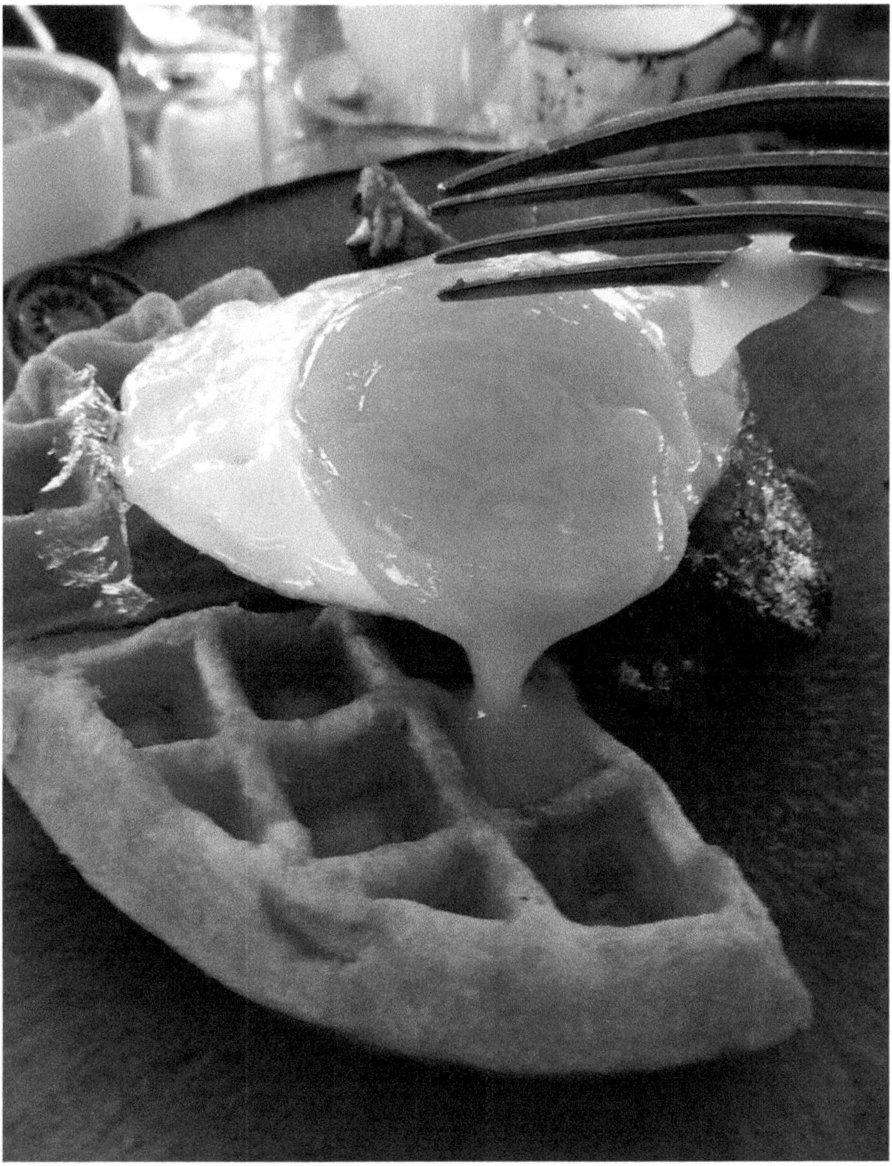

36 Mozzarella & Almond Flour Chaffles

Servings: 2

Cooking Time: 8 Minutes

Ingredients:

- ½ cup Mozzarella cheese, shredded
- 1 large organic egg
- 2 tablespoons blanched almond flour
- ¼ teaspoon organic baking powder

Directions:

1. Preheat a mini waffle iron and then grease it.
2. In a medium bowl, place all ingredients and with a fork, mix until well combined.
3. Place half of the mixture into preheated waffle iron and cook for about 4 minutes or until golden brown.
4. Repeat with the remaining mixture.
5. Serve warm.

Nutrition Info:

perServings: Calories: 98 Net Carb: 1.4g Fat: 7.1g Saturated Fat: 1g Carbohydrates: 2.2g Dietary Fiber: 0.8g Sugar: 0.2g Protein: 7g

37 Pulled Pork Chaffle Sandwiches

Servings: 4

Cooking Time: 28 Minutes

Ingredients:

- 2 eggs, beaten
- 1 cup finely grated cheddar cheese
- ¼ tsp baking powder
- 2 cups cooked and shredded pork
- 1 tbsp sugar-free BBQ sauce
- 2 cups shredded coleslaw mix
- 2 tbsp apple cider vinegar
- ½ tsp salt
- ¼ cup ranch dressing

Directions:

1. Preheat the waffle iron.
2. In a medium bowl, mix the eggs, cheddar cheese, and baking powder.

3. Open the iron and add a quarter of the mixture. Close and cook until crispy, 7 minutes.
4. Transfer the chaffle to a plate and make 3 more chaffles in the same manner.
5. Meanwhile, in another medium bowl, mix the pulled pork with the BBQ sauce until well combined. Set aside.
6. Also, mix the coleslaw mix, apple cider vinegar, salt, and ranch dressing in another medium bowl.
7. When the chaffles are ready, on two pieces, divide the pork and then top with the ranch coleslaw. Cover with the remaining chaffles and insert mini skewers to secure the sandwiches.
8. Enjoy afterward.

Nutrition Info:

perServings: Calories 374Fats 23.61gCarbs 8.2gNet Carbs 8.2gProtein 28.05g

38 Cheddar & Egg White Chaffles

Servings: 4

Cooking Time: 12 Minutes

Ingredients:

- 2 egg whites
- 1 cup Cheddar cheese, shredded

Directions:

1. Preheat a mini waffle iron and then grease it.
2. In a small bowl, place the egg whites and cheese and stir to combine.
3. Place ¼ of the mixture into preheated waffle iron and cook for about 4 minutes or until golden brown.
4. Repeat with the remaining mixture.
5. Serve warm.

Nutrition Info:

perServings: Calories: 122Net Carb: 0.5gFat: 9.4gSaturated Fat: Carbohydrates: 0.5gDietary Fiber: 0g Sugar: 0.3gProtein: 8.8g

39 Spicy Shrimp And Chaffles

Servings: 4

Cooking Time: 31 Minutes

Ingredients:

- For the shrimp:
- 1 tbsp olive oil
- 1 lb jumbo shrimp, peeled and deveined
- 1 tbsp Creole seasoning
- Salt to taste
- 2 tbsp hot sauce
- 3 tbsp butter
- 2 tbsp chopped fresh scallions to garnish
- For the chaffles:
- 2 eggs, beaten
- 1 cup finely grated Monterey Jack cheese

Directions:

1. For the shrimp:
2. Heat the olive oil in a medium skillet over medium heat.

3. Season the shrimp with the Creole seasoning and salt. Cook in the oil until pink and opaque on both sides, 2 minutes.
4. Pour in the hot sauce and butter. Mix well until the shrimp is adequately coated in the sauce, 1 minute.
5. Turn the heat off and set aside.
6. For the chaffles:
7. Preheat the waffle iron.
8. In a medium bowl, mix the eggs and Monterey Jack cheese.
9. Open the iron and add a quarter of the mixture. Close and cook until crispy, 7 minutes.
10. Transfer the chaffle to a plate and make 3 more chaffles in the same manner.
11. Cut the chaffles into quarters and place on a plate.
12. Top with the shrimp and garnish with the scallions.
13. Serve warm.

Nutrition Info:

perServings: Calories 342Fats 19.75gCarbs 2.8gNet Carbs 2.3gProtein 36.01g

40 Creamy Chicken Chaffle Sandwich

Servings: 2

Cooking Time: 10 Minutes

Ingredients:

- Cooking spray
- 1 cup chicken breast fillet, cubed
- Salt and pepper to taste
- ¼ cup all-purpose cream
- 4 garlic chaffles
- Parsley, chopped

Directions:

1. Spray your pan with oil.
2. Put it over medium heat.
3. Add the chicken fillet cubes.
4. Season with salt and pepper.
5. Reduce heat and add the cream.
6. Spread chicken mixture on top of the chaffle.
7. Garnish with parsley and top with another chaffle.

Nutrition Info:

perServings: Calories 273Total Fat 34g Saturated Fat 4.1g Cholesterol 62mg Sodium 373mg Total Carbohydrate 22.5g Dietary Fiber 1.1g Total Sugars 3.2g Protein 17.5g Potassium 177mg

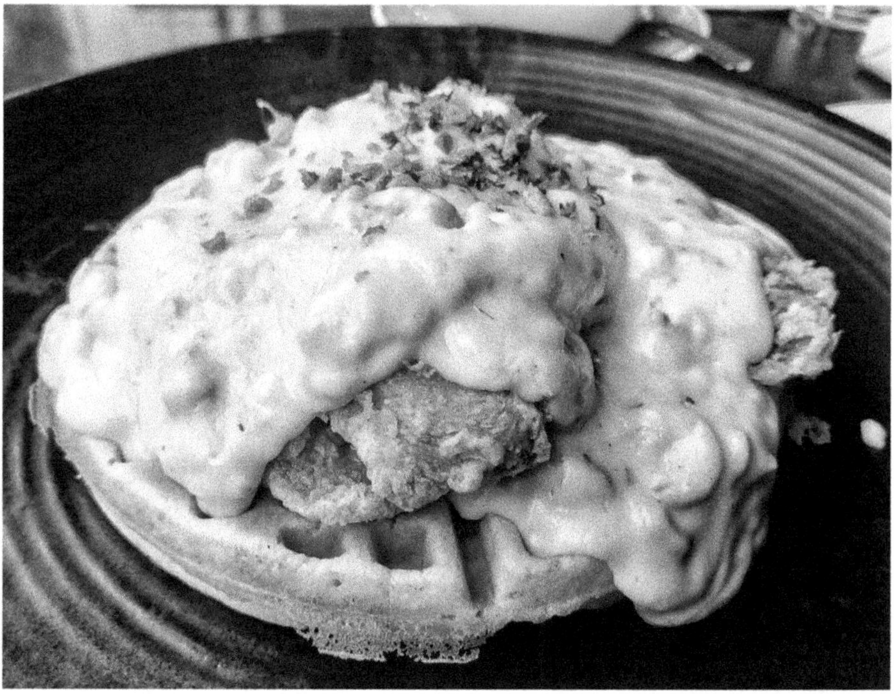

41 Chaffle Cannoli

Servings: 4

Cooking Time: 28 Minutes

Ingredients:

- For the chaffles:
- 1 large egg
- 1 egg yolk
- 3 tbsp butter, melted
- 1 tbso swerve confectioner's
- 1 cup finely grated Parmesan cheese
- 2 tbsp finely grated mozzarella cheese
- For the cannoli filling:
- ½ cup ricotta cheese
- 2 tbsp swerve confectioner's sugar
- 1 tsp vanilla extract
- 2 tbsp unsweetened chocolate chips for garnishing

Directions:

1. Preheat the waffle iron.
2. Meanwhile, in a medium bowl, mix all the ingredients for the chaffles.
3. Open the iron, pour in a quarter of the mixture, cover, and cook until crispy, 7 minutes.
4. Remove the chaffle onto a plate and make 3 more with the remaining batter.
5. Meanwhile, for the cannoli filling:
6. Beat the ricotta cheese and swerve confectioner's sugar until smooth. Mix in the vanilla.
7. On each chaffle, spread some of the filling and wrap over.
8. Garnish the creamy ends with some chocolate chips.
9. Serve immediately.

Nutrition Info:

perServings: Calories 308Fats 25.05gCarbs 5.17gNet Carbs 5.17gProtein 15.18g

42 Strawberry Shortcake Chaffle Bowls

Servings: 4

Cooking Time: 28 Minutes

Ingredients:

- 1 egg, beaten
- ½ cup finely grated mozzarella cheese
- 1 tbsp almond flour
- ¼ tsp baking powder
- 2 drops cake batter extract
- 1 cup cream cheese, softened
- 1 cup fresh strawberries, sliced
- 1 tbsp sugar-free maple syrup

Directions:

1. Preheat a waffle bowl maker and grease lightly with cooking spray.
2. Meanwhile, in a medium bowl, whisk all the ingredients except the cream cheese and strawberries.
3. Open the iron, pour in half of the mixture, cover, and cook until crispy, 6 to 7 minutes.

4. Remove the chaffle bowl onto a plate and set aside.
5. Make a second chaffle bowl with the remaining batter.
6. To serve, divide the cream cheese into the chaffle bowls and top with the strawberries.
7. Drizzle the filling with the maple syrup and serve.

Nutrition Info:

perServings: Calories 235Fats 20.62gCarbs 5.9gNet Carbs 5gProtein 7.51g

43 Chocolate Melt Chaffles

Servings: 4

Cooking Time: 36 Minutes

Ingredients:

- For the chaffles:
- 2 eggs, beaten
- ¼ cup finely grated Gruyere cheese
- 2 tbsp heavy cream
- 1 tbsp coconut flour
- 2 tbsp cream cheese, softened
- 3 tbsp unsweetened cocoa powder
- 2 tsp vanilla extract
- A pinch of salt
- For the chocolate sauce:
- 1/3 cup + 1 tbsp heavy cream
- 1 ½ oz unsweetened baking chocolate, chopped
- 1 ½ tsp sugar-free maple syrup
- 1 ½ tsp vanilla extract

Directions:

1. For the chaffles:
2. Preheat the waffle iron.
3. In a medium bowl, mix all the ingredients for the chaffles.
4. Open the iron and add a quarter of the mixture. Close and cook until crispy, 7 minutes.
5. Transfer the chaffle to a plate and make 3 more with the remaining batter.
6. For the chocolate sauce:
7. Pour the heavy cream into saucepan and simmer over low heat, 3 minutes.
8. Turn the heat off and add the chocolate. Allow melting for a few minutes and stir until fully melted, 5 minutes.
9. Mix in the maple syrup and vanilla extract.
10. Assemble the chaffles in layers with the chocolate sauce sandwiched between each layer.
11. Slice and serve immediately.

Nutrition Info:

perServings: Calories 172Fats 13.57gCarbs 6.65gNet Carbs 3.65gProtein 5.76g

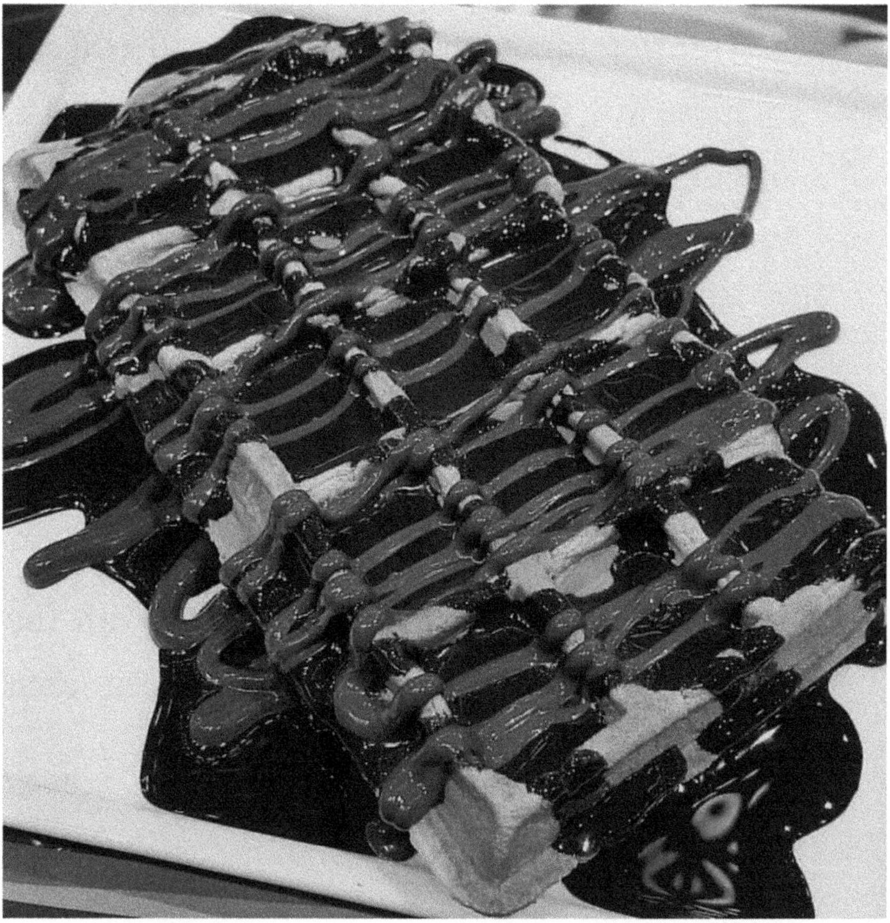

44 Pumpkin & Pecan Chaffle

Servings: 2

Cooking Time: 10 Minutes

Ingredients:

- 1 egg, beaten
- ½ cup mozzarella cheese, grated
- ½ teaspoon pumpkin spice
- 1 tablespoon pureed pumpkin
- 2 tablespoons almond flour
- 1 teaspoon sweetener
- 2 tablespoons pecans, chopped

Directions:

1. Turn on the waffle maker.
2. Beat the egg in a bowl.
3. Stir in the rest of the ingredients.
4. Pour half of the mixture into the device.
5. Seal the lid.
6. Cook for 5 minutes.
7. Remove the chaffle carefully.
8. Repeat the steps to make the second chaffle.

Nutrition Info:

perServings: Calories 210Total Fat 17 g Saturated Fat 10 g Cholesterol 110 mg Sodium 250 mg Potassium 570 mgTotal Carbohydrate 4.6 g Dietary Fiber 1.7 g Protein 11 g Total Sugars 2 g

45 Spicy Jalapeno & Bacon Chaffles

Servings:2

Cooking Time: 5 Minutes

Ingredients:

- 1 oz. cream cheese
- 1 large egg
- 1/2 cup cheddar cheese
- 2 tbsps. bacon bits
- 1/2 tbsp. jalapenos
- 1/4 tsp baking powder

Directions:

1. Switch on your waffle maker.
2. Grease your waffle maker with cooking spray and let it heat up.
3. Mix together egg and vanilla extract in a bowl first.
4. Add baking powder, jalapenos and bacon bites.
5. Add in cheese last and mix together.

6. Pour the chaffles batter intothe maker and cook the chaffles for about 2-3 minutesutes.
7. Once chaffles are cooked, remove from the maker.
8. Serve hot and enjoy!

Nutrition Info:

perServings: Protein: 24% 5kcal Fat: 70% 175 kcal Carbohydrates: 6% 15 kcal

46 Zucchini Parmesan Chaffles

Servings: 2

Cooking Time: 14 Minutes

Ingredients:

- 1 cup shredded zucchini
- 1 egg, beaten
- ½ cup finely grated Parmesan cheese
- Salt and freshly ground black pepper to taste

Directions:

1. Preheat the waffle iron.
2. Put all the ingredients in a medium bowl and mix well.
3. Open the iron and add half of the mixture. Close and cook until crispy, 7 minutes.
4. Remove the chaffle onto a plate and make another with the remaining mixture.
5. Cut each chaffle into wedges and serve afterward.

Nutrition Info:

perServings: Calories 138Fats 9.07gCarbs 3.81gNet Carbs 3.71gProtein 10.02g

47 Cheddar & Almond Flour Chaffles

Servings: 2

Cooking Time: 10 Minutes

Ingredients:

- 1 large organic egg, beaten
- ½ cup Cheddar cheese, shredded
- 2 tablespoons almond flour

Directions:

1. Preheat a mini waffle iron and then grease it.
2. In a bowl, place the egg, Cheddar cheese and almond flour and beat until well combined.
3. Place half of the mixture into preheated waffle iron and cook for about 5 minutes or until golden brown.
4. Repeat with the remaining mixture.
5. Serve warm.

Nutrition Info:

perServings: Calories: 195Net Carb: 1gFat: 15.Saturated Fat: 7gCarbohydrates: 1.8gDietary Fiber: 0.8g Sugar: 0.6gProtein: 10.2g

48 Simple& Beginner Chaffle

Servings:2

Cooking Time: 5 Minutes

Ingredients:

- 1 large egg
- 1/2 cup mozzarella cheese, shredded
- Cooking spray

Directions:

1. Switch on your waffle maker.
2. Beat the egg with a fork in a small mixing bowl.
3. Once the egg is beaten, add the mozzarella and mix well.
4. Spray the waffle makerwith cooking spray.
5. Pour the chaffles mixture in a preheated waffle maker and let it cook for about 2-3 minutes.
6. Once the chaffles are cooked, carefully remove them from the maker and cook the remaining batter.

7. Serve hot with coffee and enjoy!

Nutrition Info:

perServings: Protein: 36% 42 kcal Fat: 60% 71 kcal Carbohydrates: 4% 5 kcal

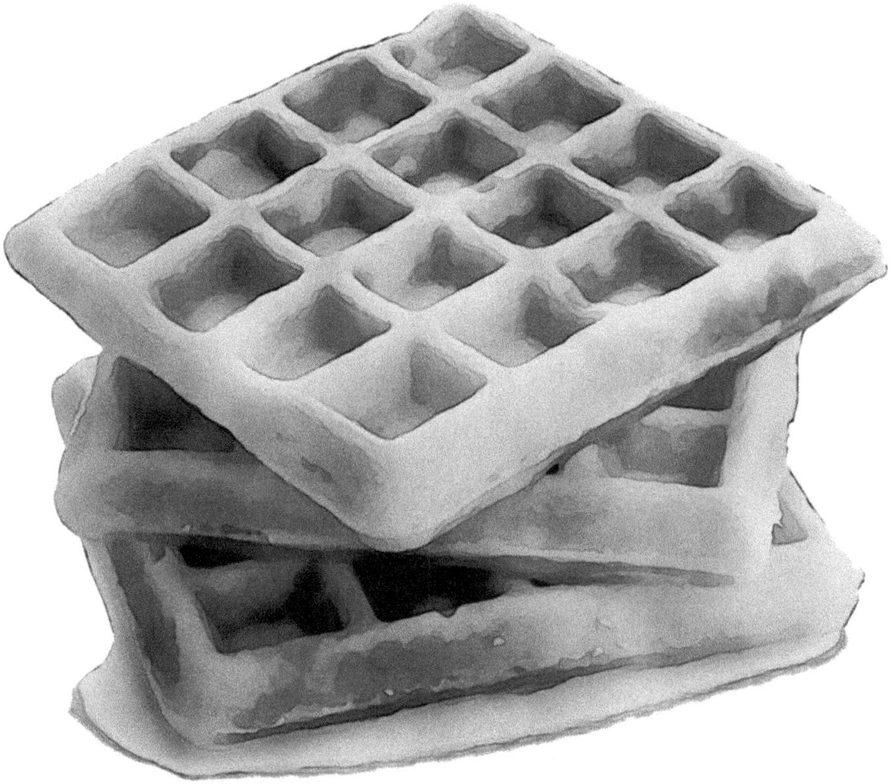

49 Asian Cauliflower Chaffles

Servings: 4

Cooking Time: 28 Minutes

Ingredients:

- For the chaffles:
- 1 cup cauliflower rice, steamed
- 1 large egg, beaten
- Salt and freshly ground black pepper to taste
- 1 cup finely grated Parmesan cheese
- 1 tsp sesame seeds
- ¼ cup chopped fresh scallions
- For the dipping sauce:
- 3 tbsp coconut aminos
- 1 ½ tbsp plain vinegar
- 1 tsp fresh ginger puree
- 1 tsp fresh garlic paste
- 3 tbsp sesame oil
- 1 tsp fish sauce
- 1 tsp red chili flakes

Directions:

1. Preheat the waffle iron.
2. In a medium bowl, mix the cauliflower rice, egg, salt, black pepper, and Parmesan cheese.
3. Open the iron and add a quarter of the mixture. Close and cook until crispy, 7 minutes.
4. Transfer the chaffle to a plate and make 3 more chaffles in the same manner.
5. Meanwhile, make the dipping sauce.
6. In a medium bowl, mix all the ingredients for the dipping sauce.
7. Plate the chaffles, garnish with the sesame seeds and scallions and serve with the dipping sauce.

Nutrition Info:

perServings: Calories 231Fats 188gCarbs 6.32gNet Carbs 5.42gProtein 9.66g

50 Sharp Cheddar Chaffles

Servings: 2

Cooking Time: 10 Minutes

Ingredients:

- 1 organic egg, beaten
- ½ cup sharp Cheddar cheese, shredded

Directions:

1. Preheat a mini waffle iron and then grease it.
2. In a small bowl, place the egg and cheese and stir to combine.
3. Place half of the mixture into preheated waffle iron and cook for about 5 minutes or until golden brown.
4. Repeat with the remaining mixture.
5. Serve warm.

Nutrition Info:

perServings**:** Calories: 145Net Carb: 0.5gFat: 11.Saturated Fat: 6.6gCarbohydrates: 0.5gDietary Fiber: 0g Sugar: 0.3gProtein: 9.8g

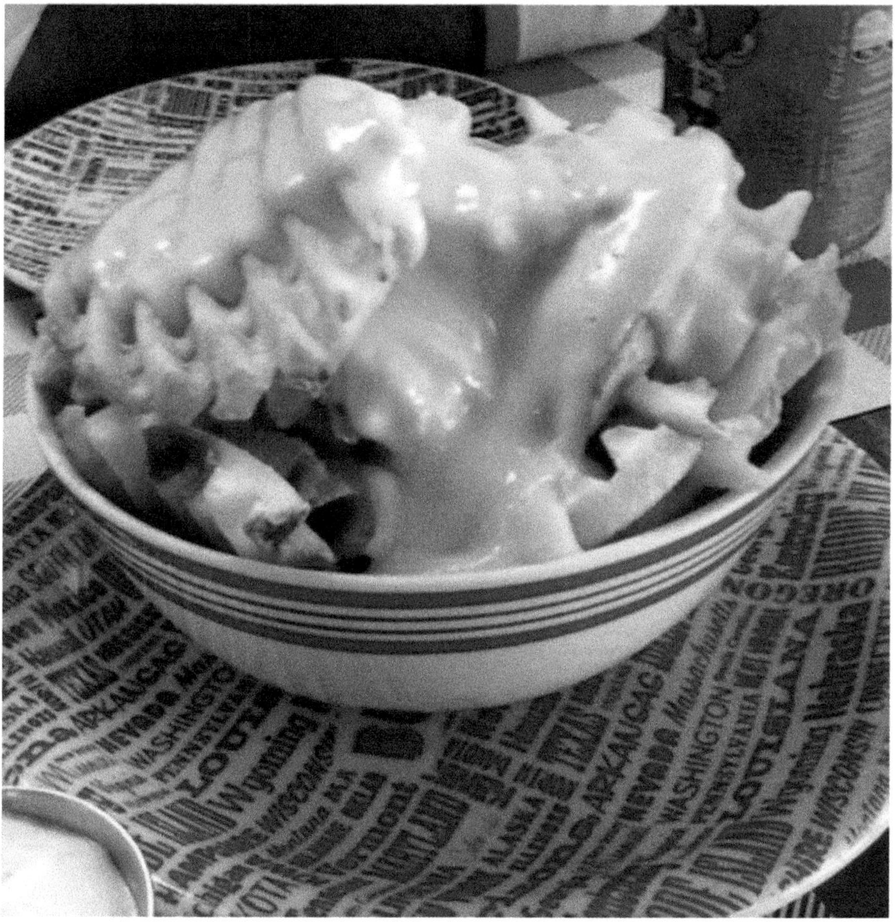
WASHINGTON
TEXAS

Lightning Source UK Ltd.
Milton Keynes UK
UKHW020642210621
385885UK00001B/24

9 781802 778281

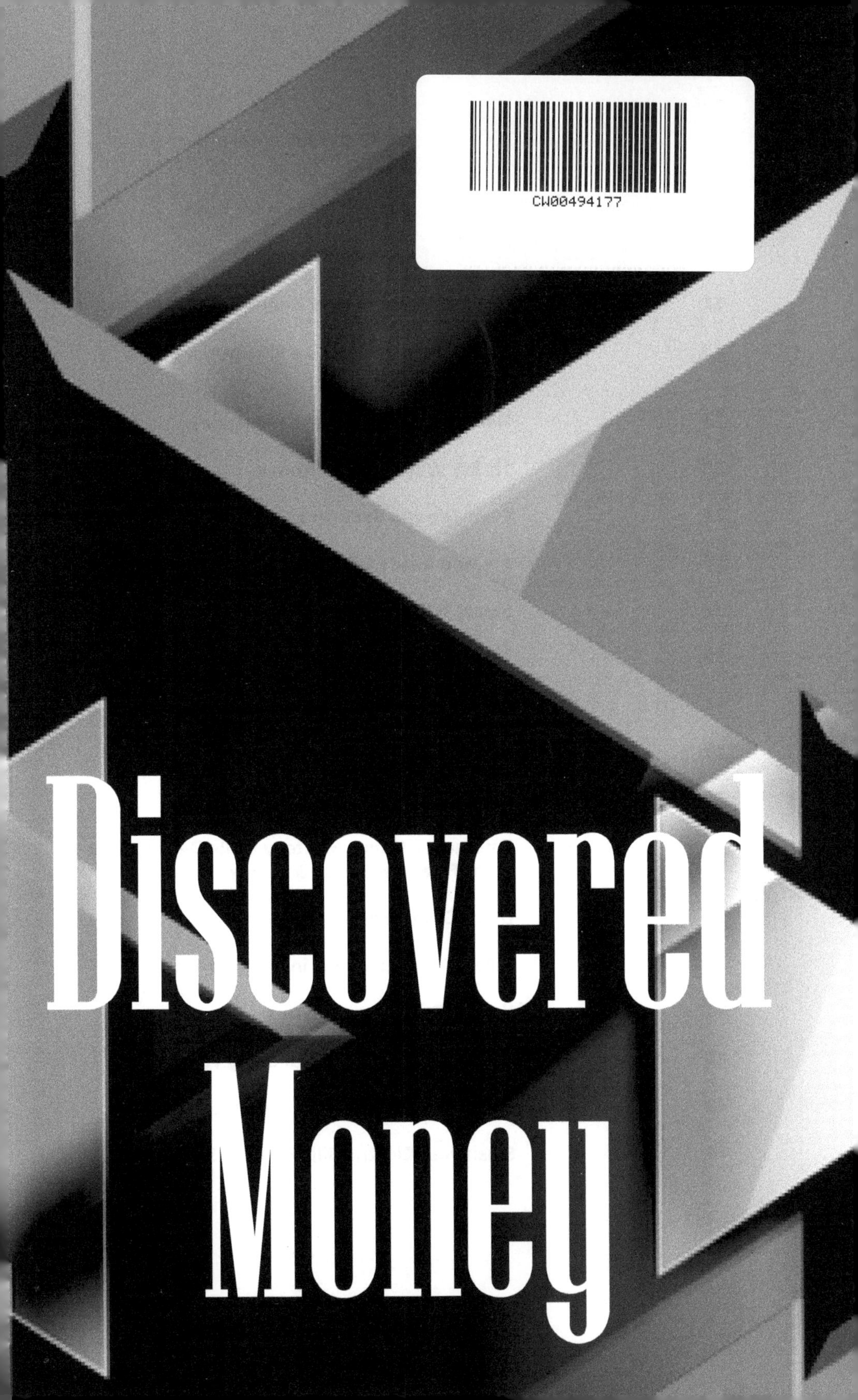

Discovered Money

Introduction

At least once in every person's life comes a time when the need is great and the resources are few. It can be hard enough to make ends meet on a decent wage, but, when the times get tough and the money just is not there to meet the need, a person can easily despair.

101 Ways to Raise Emergency Money has been written with you in mind. If you are forever trying to come up with inventive ways to earn and save more then this creative ebook will absolutely thrill you.

When a person can have good financial control and a good plan of action. Should emergency funds be needed, a person can then sleep better at night. There is no real magic formula for coming up with on-the-spot emergency cash. There is a good deal of thinking through and the putting of a good plan into action. If you can do that, you have it made. That is truly all that any one of us can do to secure out tomorrows.

How to Cope with a Cash Crisis

If you are hit with a serious money crisis and you find yourself scrambling around for emergency money, here's how to assess your situation and get back on your feet.

All of a sudden and without warning, your roof begins to leak! Your hot water heater shuts down and your computer goes up in smoke, the clutch needs to be replaced in your car and your son decides to have his wedding on the Isle of Oahu - all of this within the same week!

As you sit, stunned and you ponder an exit strategy you receive a friendly letter from the IRS explaining that you miscalculated your taxes in 1996, and they now own your house.

This Kind of Money Emergency Requires your Immediate Attention
What do you do?

The above scenario looks like a money emergency of biblical proportions. You are afraid to open your front door for fear of finding a swarm of locusts!

Thank goodness, there are things you can still do to restore your financial life and equilibrium—and perhaps even fend off future misfortune—without having to sell your very soul.

Learning to Cope with a Money Emergency

Wherever there are money woes, you can be sure to find crippling emotional setback. Avoid it all you try, you might just as well begin to prepare for the devastating fiscal and the emotional fallout that is sure to come. You will need to cope very well with both if you hope to make a solid financial comeback.

Whenever a money emergency hits, it will be your ability to deal with the individual pitfalls that will hold you in good stead. It is when a series of financial hits come your way that the stress will tend to accumulate and make your life much more difficult to cope.

You will not be so overwhelmed when you can calmly and rationally look at each individual problem as it arises. If you sit back wringing your hands with worry and allow all of your emergencies to pile into one; you will find yourself down for the count.

Calm must take center stage. You must NEVER allow yourself the luxury of panic. There is no one there for you to just take over. You are all you have.

The more you panic, the less effective you will be. You need to keep a very clear head to be able to sit down and come up with an appropriate plan. Be aware of your own tendency to sabotage your plans further. It is only when you are at your most calm that you will be prepared to get to where you need to be and then overcome.

Being Calm is the First Key to Managing a Money Emergency

At even the first hint of a money emergency, it's important not to act right away. If you do you will inevitably make a mistake! First, before you can manage your finances again, you have to first manage your emotions. You absolutely must regain your balance before you can even begin to make a plan.

If your money emergency demands that you act quickly, think first about seeking the advice of a debt counselor, money coach or financial planner. Whenever possible think about seeking out the aid of a financially perceptive friend or family member who can help you to come to a clearer perspective.

Remember the old adage that "two heads are always better than just one!" You won't need to make a major cash investment if you're strapped. Look for a planner who will give you a one-hour consultation for $150. Often times this will be all you will need to securely turn the corner.

Time to Crunch some Numbers

The first step toward establishing financial stability is to step back, take a deep breath and assess the damage. Possibly one of the bigger mistakes people make when they're in a financial crisis is not being prepared to make a clear assessment of where they're at.

You can easily become overwhelmed. However, totaling up the damage serves two important purposes. First, you need to know exactly how much you owe, how much money you have in hand and what it will take to cover the distance between the two. Second, you will want to avoid any other mishaps, such as penalties, further repairs, missed deadlines, etc.

If you are not properly prepared, you must become prepared on the spot. Any type of money crisis will catch you unaware and you will feel cornered. Wouldn't it be ideal to be ready and waiting for the crisis? How likely is this to happen to you, though?

Most people will be at least somewhat prepared. If the crisis is not too dire, they will be able to handle it ok. Some will be sunk from the get go. The idea is to not be overwhelmed and to have a good plan of action, no matter how little or how a lot. You need to be entirely prepared to deal with any sized setback.

Ideally, those unexpected expenses could be covered by the funds in the Irregular Expenses account in any good budget. Unfortunately, though, there is always a common problem. You might well have an emergency stash—but it's most often depleted. This same problem affects the majority of us so take heart.

At about this time many people make the mistake of turning to plastic for relief. Resist this one. You will only be transferring your problems from one pocket to the other.

On the other hand, if you are sure you can handle using credit cards to deal with a cash emergency, you had better be sure you could pay them off when the time comes. Otherwise, why add yet another debt and another problem. Eventually, it will all catch up with you.

If you're truly running while on your last leg, consider taking out a home equity line of credit. This will work for some. The interest is tax deductible, but those aren't fixed rates. Be smart about this remedy, though. Unless you plan to pay back the amount you borrowed promptly, it can end up costing you more than you thought—especially if you've already depleted your own equity.

The Idea is to Make a Smart Decision and not a Rash one

Think well before borrowing from your 401(k) or IRA. There are loopholes that allow you to do so, but there are also hidden costs—never mind potential taxes, penalties and other consequences. Keep in mind that if you were to lose your job, you'd have to repay the loan immediately, or be taxed as though it was a withdrawal. This remedy could be very costly in the long run.

Increase your Cash Flow without Going Further into Debt

- Take on a hobby that you can translate into dollars. Can you walk a neighborhood dog? Teach basket weaving? Host a dining room? Baby-sit for your sister's kids? Do Computer graphics? Consider which of your talents might be worth a few extra bucks and then go out there and do it.

- Take on a part-time job. The holidays are soon coming up, and many people supplement their salaries with part-time retail jobs. Just don't spend it all on holiday gifts and be sure to bank it into your savings.

- Spend more wisely. We all have our own ways of wasting money. Now see how you can eliminate the ones that you wouldn't miss. Just saving the dollar you would normally spend on that cup of coffee each day adds up.

- Borrow from a trusted friend or relative. The interest rate is low to nil, the cash is quick—but guilt is even higher. Be sure you have a plan for how you're going to pay back the loan even before you approach them.

Nowhere to go but up

You can spend your precious time crying in your milk wondering why you have been singled out in this way or you can get busy and look at how this could have happened to you in the first place. You will need to face some touch answers if you want to avoid future financial crises.

Suffering a serious financial crisis is an excellent time to self-assess. Ask yourself where you went wrong, where you're not paying attention—and how you might be setting yourself up for future financial setbacks. Understanding the answers to these important questions will help you out next time around should the same befall you.

Be prepared before the crisis starts. You won't be able to anticipate every time a financial burden lands in your lap, but, if you want to be cushioned against it, you have to anticipate the unanticipated.

Be very careful. An emergency fund is set up for . . . emergencies. It's not supposed to be depleted on a whim and every month. Take a closer look at your expenses these last few months, and if you have had to lean heavily on your emergency account to pad your budget, it's time to rethink your money management issues and in a hurry.

Pay special attention. Take a page out of this lady's book...she noticed that her towels were slightly singed when she took them out of the dryer one day. Instead of calling the repair guy, she shrugged it off—until the next load caused her entire house to go up in flames. We all have these same moments where we glimpse a potential crisis hovering on the horizon and do nothing until it is all too late. Pay attention to the smaller details and avoid the larger calamities.

Plan further ahead. Your clutch is likely going to give out every 80,000 miles or so. The roof can give out every 15 to 20 years. A vacuum cleaner might give up the dust in as much as five. Avoid the obvious and pay excessively later. It is your call.

Your five-year-old desktop is getting creaky. You could wait until it dies. However, according to Murphy's Law of Money, it will expire at the worst possible moment. Either way, paying for a new computer might not be part of the budget so planning ahead gives you some control over when you take the hit. Start to plan today for what you know will be coming—come hell or high water. Plan smartly for the inevitable.

Start to Build your Emergency Fund

Finding money during an emergency can be very difficult if you fail to plan. Establish emergency savings in both good times and in bad. The chance is very good that you will be called upon to put out a sum of money on the spot and when you least expect it.

It is a very good rule of thumb to sock away three to six months' living expenses. You can also use this same money when you're faced with major, unplanned expenses such as a car that breaks down or much needed college funds.

The purpose of this type of savings plan is to put the money away consistently, and then tap into it for true emergencies. The success of this type of long-range savings plan will depend less on the rate of return than on, day-by-day, putting the money away and then leaving it there for a true emergency.

Lock it away and then hide the key.

People who are living on a fixed-income will have the toughest time setting aside money for emergencies. If you can manage to just squeeze out another

$10 or $20 each month and sock it away into a money market account, it's worth doing.

If you decide you need $2,000 in an emergency fund, look at what you can afford to sacrifice each month from your current budget and then look at that sum of money as a bill to pay yourself. Decide on a monthly amount and then put that same amount aside every month and then watch it grow. Once you have reached your goal of $2,000 you'll now be in the habit of putting away that extra set amount each month. Keep on doing it.

Financial planners echo the idea of treating your emergency fund as a bill. Put the money away each month, but don't be tempted by the latest sale. You are not to touch the amount, except for in an emergency.

Putting money aside on your own is hard. Retirement plans are successful because the money comes out of your paycheck before you can get your hands on it and because there are taxes and penalties for early withdrawals.

Stashing money away in an easy access money market account takes discipline. Limit your access to the emergency fund. You can have immediate access to some of the money, but not all of it. The bulk of the fund is to be used, strictly, for emergencies and nothing else.

Once you have saved up about two months of living expenses, move one month of expenses to a one-month CD. When the CD matures, roll the principal and interest into another one-month CD. Your savings will grow well this way.

As you continue making regular payments to the emergency fund money market account, you will soon have another month of living expenses that can be used to invest in a two-or three-month CD. If you are wishing to set aside six months of expenses, continue the process until you can comfortably purchase a six-month CD. Your savings will accumulate quickly this way.

Building your Emergency Fund

Before you start stashing away your money for an emergency, the first step in building your emergency fund is to figure out just how much money you have to put aside in the first place.

People often don't know where they're spending their money. Once you can account for every penny, it's a lot easier to decide where you can cut back and start to save.

You can't always account for emergencies so it is more critical to build the fund as fast as possible.

Say Good-bye to Credit Cards

One of the best ways to save money the fastest is to clip up all of those expensive credit cards.

Credit cards are perhaps one of the most expensive forms of money. A very good rule of thumb is, unless you pay off your credit card bills each month, don't use the cards for anything you can either eat or wear.

Another good rule of thumb is to consolidate your debt. If you have several credit cards, each at different rates of interest, why not fold them into a home equity loan and then write off the interest payments? This is a good way to begin an emergency savings fund.

Here are some good suggestions for budget trimming that can work for just about everyone:

When mortgage rates are especially low—consider refinancing your mortgage and, while you're at it, your car loans, too.

When you live in an area that has good public transportation, see if you can get by on one car instead of two.

Make your current car last. With good maintenance, you will be able to replace it every six to eight years instead of every three years.

Do a periodical energy check on the house. Replace all essentials such as cracked storm windows and renew the weather stripping.

Cancel subscriptions to magazines or newspapers that you're not reading.

Eat out less often and learn to be creative using leftovers. If you stop for a morning cup of coffee at the local Deli, make coffee at home.

For the kids weekly allowance cut it back. Explain to them that every member of the family needs to contribute to the emergency fund for it to work.

Remember, too, that you will be teaching your kids to be frugal and to develop good spending habits.

Saving money on your own brings many rewards, and like most other things, it becomes easier over time. In the end, your entire family will have peace of mind that comes from knowing you have financial resources set up and ready for when times are the toughest. The sacrifices you make now will be realized when you need the most comfort as a family.

Painless Ways to Find Money for an Emergency

If your plan for money for your next emergency is to scoop up the change that falls between the cushions, you might want to come up with a plan to add to that stash. It is always a good idea to have a little extra green for the lean times. Rainy days could be just around the corner. Rainy day funds become necessary! Here are some very clever and virtually painless ways to put aside some money now!

Put aside a large envelope, cookie tin, coffee jar or something similar. At the end of every week, throw a couple of dollars aside. By the end of your first month you should have some extra cash put aside to have a nice start on an emergency fund. The idea to doing this is don't count it or spend it. Place it somewhere that is hidden away. Put it somewhere that you won't be tempted to dip into it. This kind of money really adds up!

The next time you treat yourself or your family to a meal out, tip yourself! Just as you go to tip the waitress 15 to 20 percent, put the same amount aside for yourself. When you get home, stash it away in your cookie jar. Every time you go through a fast food window, put a dollar away for that cookie jar, too!

The next time you get a good raise, instead of applying it to your cost of living, bank it! This way you will always be living one raise behind and your bank account will be growing by some 3 percent.

Take advantage of that cash back option! Next time you make a purchase using your debit card, ask for a small amount of cash back. Instead of spending it, stash it away in your cookie jar! Chances are you won't even miss that extra $1, $2 or $5 bill and come emergency time, you will notice how the amount has piled up.

Next time you pay off that big-ticket item like a new car or tuition, continue to make the payments to yourself! Set up a savings account and each month slip the ghost payment into it. Watch as it builds nicely.

If you have noticed that you can get a better long distance telephone plan and you want to switch, allocate the savings to your cookie jar. You won't likely miss that little bit of extra money, and you will have a better telephone plan, too.

Consider joining a Christmas club. You will save a lot of money. Each year you put aside a bit of money and place it into a hamper program. Then, as Christmas rolls around you don't need to scramble looking for Christmas cheer to share with your family. Your hamper arrives filled to the brim with all kinds of seasonal goodies that you paid for over the previous year. You can easily put aside $50 each year towards your emergency fund this way and you and your family will enjoy a hassle free Christmas.

Sign up for a grocery shopping membership card. At the bottom of your store receipt, you will see a print out that states how much you save each week. It really adds up. You can easily save an average of $15 on each weekly grocery trip. Add that amount, each week, to your savings cookie jar.

Did you enjoy your tax refund this year? Sure you did, we all did. That's because of the new tax laws. Many people will have a little extra money coming their way after April 15. Decide to deposit that extra money right away into your savings account or cash it and then stash it. Sure you can come up with plenty of ways you can use that money now, but put it away for later. You might need it even more later.

If you are a responsible spender, take out a credit card that rewards your loyalty. When you pay off the bill every month, use a card that promises a cash reward and bank the money. Use your reward credit card smartly and you could end up with a very nice windfall for your rainy day fund.

Put aside a large mouthed jar in the kitchen. It is very likely that your parents and grandparents had one. At the end of each workday simply empty your pockets or clean out your change purse. All the change goes into the jar. Who wants to carry around all that dead weight, anyway? Your spare change adds up a lot faster than you think. While you are at it, add at least one bill to your change jar at the end of each week. Aim for a $20!

Is it time to give up that nasty smoking habit? Imagine the money you will save! If you are not quite ready to quit at least cut back by half. Put the savings each day into your change jar and watch it overflow!

Convert to a coin-operated laundry. Keep a jar on your washer and dryer and every time you go to do a load of laundry, slip in a coin or two. This adds up month by month.

The next time you go to return a movie rental on time, pay yourself the late fee. You will see how quickly that $1.50 to $4 can add up.

If you yearn to loose some weight, try rewarding yourself the cost of the item that you do without each day. Put that money into your change jar. You will look great and you will be saving for a rainy day!

Place a large jar by the telephone. Everyone must drop in a coin to make a call. All proceeds go to the emergency fund. This one works!

Emergencies always crop up. They are always guaranteed, unlike the money to deal with them. Be prepared and plan!

Every Day Ways to Save Money for an Emergency

When you think about it, there are a good many ways to save those precious pennies. Some ways will require some sacrifice, while others will require little before thought.

The point is to be forever mindful of saving those extra pennies and before you know it, you will have saved up a tidy sum.

- Spend less money than you earn each week.
- Seek out a higher paying job.
- Keep your job skills sharp and up-to-date so that when a new opportunity comes up, you will be on your toes and first in line.
- Adjust your lifestyle to always spend a bit less.
- Create a firm financial budget to encourage saving.
- If you must use credit cards/cut up those you can do without.
- If you must use credit cards, pay them all down in full each month.
- If you have credit card debt at high rates, consolidate at once.
- Figure out a way to lower your student loan payments.
- Just say NO to spending money whenever possible.
- Lower your expenses, one by one.
- Stop purchasing items that you can do without.
- Forego purchasing non-essential items.
- Refinance your mortgage or debt at a much lower rate.
- Refinance your car loan at a much lower interest rate.

- Find cheaper insurance rates/then switch over.
- Use coupons to shop with. Don't purchase without a discount coupon.
- Wait for things to first go on sale before buying. Take advantage of catalog saving certificates.
- Don't buy an item just because it is on sale.
- Buy generic or non-name brand merchandise as much as possible.
- Wait for prices to fall to a discounted rate before buying (applies especially to electronics items).
- Reward yourself for saving money. Enjoy as your debt shrinks and your investments grow.
- Drive used cars or leases rather than brand new cars.
- Reduce your auto insurance.
- Don't eat out as much as you'd like to.
- If you do eat out, buy gift certificates for half price meals.
- Buy only discount magazines.
- Do more stay in activities at home.
- Invest the money you save to earn even more.
- Create a plan to save $200 each month (as much as you can manage.) Never miss the monthly savings payment to yourself and try to find ways to increase it.
- Don't spend money just because you have it.
- Look into getting a better quality education.
- Stay very busy – you will have less time to spend money.

- Find an interesting hobby to occupy your time and stop you from spending money.
- Find a hobby that you can turn into earnings.
- Stop smoking and bank the savings.
- Go on a sensible diet and lose weight. You will save money on food, look and feel better, and your long-term healthcare costs should fall dramatically.
- Look carefully at how you spend and save your money.
- Learn how to manage your finances by reading financial publications.
- Increase the amount of money you earn through a second job, promotion, new job, investments, etc.
- Don't try to compete with your friends and neighbors. Be satisfied with what you have.
- Don't compare yourself to your friends and neighbors. Be happy being you.
- Sell your car and take the bus to work if you can.
- Contribute the maximum each year to your 401K or to an IRA.
- Buy Dental Insurance before you need it.
- Buy Health Insurance before you need it.
- Paying down your debt is also a way to save money (it saves you from a debt payment and brings you closer to having money to invest).
- Switch to lower your telephone bill.
- Lower your cable bill by deleting pay channels or switch to satellite.
- Earn extra money by completing short surveys online.

- Practice restraint at all times.
- Be patient when bargain shopping.
- Start saving money today!
- Don't give up -- put just $10 aside, today!

More Creative Ways to Save Money

- Shop for clothing at thrift shops (especially for young kids). Look for gently worn or even new clothes for 1/10 the price of new (or less).
- Pay your bills online. It's protected and you can save with stamps.
- Put your kids on the school bus rather than driving them to school.
- Slipcover or reupholster older furniture for a quick update rather than buying expensive new furniture.
- Refinish furniture and/or decorate with new paint. Use older and broken furniture to make a unique piece.
- Take your lunch to work every day! Make your meals in bulk and then freeze them in smaller containers to save even more money.
- Buy a bread maker to make your own bread. This is much cheaper than $2.00 a loaf, and tastes terrific!
- Shop for dented canned goods and outdated toiletries at salvage grocery stores.
- Read magazine subscriptions at the library or buy them at the thrift shop for .25 to .50 after someone else has read them.
- Stop drinking expensive sodas and make Kool-Aid or decaffeinated iced tea, instead.
- Cancel expensive telephone options like call waiting.

- Check out library books instead of buying expensive new titles.

- When you wash your hair every day don't lather twice. Saves shampoo!
- Change your eating habits and avoid expensive, processed foods.

- Exercise and eat right to keep your doctor bills down.
- Brush and floss your teeth to keep the dentist bill down.

- Keep up on regular auto maintenance and avoid costly repair.
- Mend your clothing instead of buying new clothes.

- Buy only clothing that does not require dry cleaning.
- Take care of your own nails. Avoid manicures.

- Simplify your hairstyle – wear a hairdo that doesn't require much maintenance.
- Get at least 3-6 quotes when shopping for items over $100.

- Develop self-control and simplify your life if possible.
- Buy only inexpensive, no-name drugstore cosmetics.

- Cut your dryer sheets in half.
- Buy generic over the counter medicine rather than name brand items when possible.
- Buy generic baby wipes, diapers, and formula, anything you can for the baby.

- Look for quality, name brand clothing at garage sales in more affluent neighborhoods.
- Find fashionable clothing in the sale departments of stores like the Gap and Stitches.

- Keep in fashion by finding basic colored tees and skirts and then add cheaper, trendy accessories.
- Buy baby clothes privately from someone that has an older child (one year older) than yours. You can find good quality clothing cheaper this way.
- When you get change back from a purchase put it in the piggy bank. Always give the cashier whole dollars, not the exact amount. In a few months, you will have "found" money that can be used for an emergency fund.
- You can save money by shopping for groceries in the "bulk foods" aisles in your grocery store.
- Bulk up in the wintertime. You don't need the heat above 68 degrees in the winter inside your house. Wear warm clothes and socks/slippers while in the house.
- Use all plastic bags you receive at the grocery store for trash bags.
- Some grocery stores give you a 5-cent credit per bag if you bring your own bags. Pennies add up over time.
- Instead of buying a new house, rent to own. The payments are cheaper.
- Install a water softener. It might be expensive to start up, but in the long run, you use less shampoo/conditioner on your hair and it saves your appliances (pipes, iron, washing machine, dish washer, kettle and hot water tank) from clogging up with lime scale.
- Breastfeed your children!
- Save money when shopping next time at the supermarket by remembering to check the lower items nearer to floor level as they are often much cheaper than those at eye level. Also, resist the temptation to purchase extra items at the checkout such as magazines and candy bars.
- When you receive a gift that you are sure you won't use, re-gift! The next time you will need to buy a gift - give away one of your own.
- Buy, slaughter and butcher your own cow. The average cost of the meat

is $1.00 per pound.

- Hand-pick your own fruits and vegetables in season. They are less expensive and better quality foods.

- The next time you yearn to see a movie wait to see it on DVD at the video store.

- Quick braking, cornering, and accelerating (speeding) will eat your gas up considerably. Never let your fuel needle go below a ½ tank, or fill it up when you drive it to "Empty". Nickel and diming your gas tank gets you no where fast!

Thrifty Ways to Save Money

Saving for an emergency need not be a chore when you are making a good effort to put money aside constantly. Be in a mood of saving and watch as that bank account accumulates.

- Instead of buying a new DVD, save money by trading with family and friends. Once a month do the rounds and before you know it, you will have a new library of good movies to enjoy.

- Plant a small garden each spring, with just the vegetables that you really like. Even a small effort every day can save you dollars usually spent on fresh vegetables at the produce market.

- Buy your bread and other bakery items at the local thrift bread store.

- Check your local library for the newest DVD/video releases and then rent three for $2.00 for two days.
- Read your local newspapers online.

- Search eBay for big ticket items and then save literally hundreds on computers, DVD players, etc.

- Keep track of the cost of items you buy a lot and get them at the cheapest store, like cleaning supplies at Family Dollar, pet food at Wal-Mart, etc.

- Make a conscious effort to combine tasks that require driving some place, so you will get the most out of your mileage.

- For your friends and family who do not feel slighted by this, send e-mail cards for holidays, birthdays and as thank you cards. In addition, e-mail family and friends who live far away, instead of calling long distance.

- Get rid of your monthly fee long distance service, and just use an access code when you do call, which is infrequently anyway and inexpensive.

- Decide which satellite channels you could do without, and give up a few shows you really like. You can save more than $20.00 on your monthly bill.

- When you buy vegetables, fruits and bread at the grocery store check the reduced-for-quick-sale carts and shelves first.

- Change the oil in your vehicles yourself.

- Save money when buying clothes for the following year at the end of the season / during the off season. You can get great mark down prices.

- Each evening take the spare change from your pockets or periodically clean out your purse and toss the coins aside. Never take any money back until the end of the year. Then take all of the coins to the bank and exchange them for cash. You'll be surprised to find out they've added up to $50, $100 or even $200.

- "Take care of your cents, and then your dollars will take care of themselves."

- Bike to work in good weather instead of driving to save on gas.

- Eat a few hearty vegetarian meals each week.

- Shop garage sales for a great source of household items, books, clothing, and furniture.

- Don't buy bottled water! Buy a good water-filter and drink tap water.

- By the end of each day put all of your change into an empty coffee can. Then roll coins as you watch TV or listen to the radio. This will add up to hundreds of dollars very quickly and gives you something good to do with your hands to relax.

Save money by reducing your energy costs. Energy can be the number two or three expense, along with the cost of rent or mortgage and food.

Switch every single bulb to compact florescent bulbs. They may be expensive but they last for years (no more replacements) and tend to use about 10-20% of the energy of regular bulbs. Buy one each time you make a shopping trip, starting in the high traffic areas of the house like the kitchen or stairway until you no longer have any incandescent bulbs left.

If you own your home, seriously consider switching any electric heating appliances to natural gas such as the hot water heater, furnace, stove or dryer. Electricity can be used for almost any device, and you pay a hefty premium on electricity for that. Gas is very efficient for heating devices; it heats up much quicker and wastes far less energy.

Do all of your laundry in cold water. Most modern detergents are just as effective in cold water as in hot water. Also, make sure any laundry that you do is a complete and full load - it takes the same amount of energy as a tenth of a load.

Try this trick with your dryer: Put it on for 20 minutes, and then put it on "air fluff" for 15 minutes. Your clothes are already hot with the water coming off as vapor and you'll find although it takes about 20% longer, you save about 50% of the energy costs of your dryer.

In the colder months when you need to use your furnace, turn the heat on to your desired temperature. When the furnace turns off (your house has been heated to temperature), turn the thermostat to the off position. If you feel cold, check the thermostat. If you 5 degrees below your desired temperature, turn the thermostat on again to your desired temperature.

Often furnaces will kick in and out to maintain your desired temperature, but furnaces are far more efficient when they are in the heat cycle for longer periods. You'll save about 50% on your furnace costs, even 30% over having a high-tech digital thermostat. Of course keep it completely off when you're out of the house.

If you ever leave the house for the weekend or longer, unplug everything. That alarm clock or VCR blinking or DVD on standby still take power. If you're leaving the house for a week, you will save real money by just unplugging all of these devices- and you'll protect your home from fire risks should there be a malfunction or power surge.

Keep your fridge and freezer as full as possible. The fewer airspaces in your fridge, the less time it takes for your fridge or freezer to cool the air. Don't have much money for food? Just buy a bunch of bread and throw it in the freezer, you usually can get bread cheaper when you buy it in large quantities anyway.

If you really need a magazine subscription make up a small group maybe with three people to divide the costs. Then each person can keep the magazine for one week.

Save money by throwing away any catalogs or magazines which tempt you to buy something.

Cereal can be frozen and it keeps for a very long time. Before that, we could never eat it fast enough and had to throw it away when it was stale. When you pour milk on it, you would never know that it had been frozen. I have not yet found a cereal that tasted bad from the freezer.

Don't throw away your empty bags of milk. Instead cut them open and wash them. You can use them as baggies. They also keep frozen foods fresh when used with a sealer.

Save money by preparing your grocery list by planning menus for the coming week and buy only what is on your list.

Borrow DVDs from friends and family instead of renting.

Set your washer to the shortest wash setting possible. Instead of washing your clothes for 10 minutes put it on for 5 minutes. It saves on your electric bill and on your clothes wear and tear.

Pick up the pennies, dimes and nickels found on the sidewalks or in parking lots. Add it to the jar of loose change you are saving and by the end of the year you can add this money to your emergency fund.

Foster the practice of team sports in your kids. The more time you spend with your kids playing sports, the less time and money they will spend at the shopping mall.

To save money on gas, don't fill the gas tank to the brim since the extra weight of the gasoline takes extra toll on engine power. Take out all items in the trunk which are not important to reduce vehicle weight.

Watch other peoples' budget-conscious movies. Buy your own jar of popcorn and add your own seasonings.

Turn off the heat at night and sleep with a hot water bottle. This works fine in a small apartment, because it heats up quickly. For people with larger houses, turning the heat down should work well, too.

If you must drink a specialty coffee, Espresso seems like a luxury item, but because it's ground finer, and you use less, the coffee lasts longer.

Shop eBay for things like razors, lotions, computer software, baby formula, diapers, etc. If you can plan ahead, you will save.

Each pay period set aside any amount that you have budgeted for but did not need to spend. For instance, you may have anticipated that $50 would be needed to maintain your car, but only had to spend $30. Take the "extra" $20 and put it into your savings account.

Even YOU can save while on a shoestring

Believe it or not, how much you save has little to do with how much you make and studies have proven this! It is time to put away the excuses; here's a roadmap for finding money you didn't even know you had.

That One Simple Word—Savings

When you hear that one, simple word, do you feel a deep sense of guilt? Of course you do - we all do. That is because, like most Americans, 75% of respondents said they knew that their savings, targeted for retirement, were insufficient.

That's cause for distress, perhaps, but not nearly as remarkable as the discovery that how much you save now has very little to do with how rich you are, today. This is so true in fact, that the middle-income earners managed to save less than the lower-income earners in that same study. Now this is remarkable when you think about it. Those with less saved more! What is the secret to their savings success?

For those of us who scrimp and save endlessly and with so little to show for it, these statistics are both annoying and embarrassing! It also means you have no excuse for inadequate savings.

The bottom line here is this: You just have to save, regardless! That means for every $10 you earn, you MUST sock away at least $1 in savings. Does not sound to be too difficult, right? WRONG!

UNLESS you have an iron clad savings plan, you will not save a single red cent! The trick is in the purpose and the plan!

WHAT IS YOUR EMERGENCY PLAN?

ARE YOU READY TO START A GOOD SAVINGS PLAN?

You are ready but you feel at a loss as to how you will come up with that extra money. You are already barely eking out a living. You can manage if you train yourself to think differently. That is the first part of any good plan. You have to think right. If you don't think right towards your money, you won't be able to manage it.

Your First Step: Rethink how you think about money

Saving money is a calm state of mind. Before you can even begin, you have to say NO to all of the spending—and stop thinking that you actually need all the stuff you're spending all of your hard-earned money on. Just don't spend.

That is simple enough! Say NO to all of the excuses and reasons for why you feel you MUST spend. Tell yourself, NO MORE EXCUSES, PERIOD! The very next time you want to buy something, take the $50 or $100 out of your wallet, instead and stash it away somewhere. Do you see the logic? That's why you call saving. You don't end up with stuff; you end up with the hard-earned MONEY.

Another new way of thinking will be to think of frugality as your savior. Become a confirmed cheapskate and do as your most frugal friends do. Pay special note to the fact that frugal friends fix the shower curtain instead of buying a new one. Sit down with Depression-era relatives and ask about how they made ends meet despite even desperate times. You want to learn to economize.

The next step in rethinking is to become inspired. Spend all of your spare time online and search out those frugal Web sites. Look at "living cheaply," "frugal living" and "voluntary simplicity." You'll find a ton of good Web sites devoted to living on less, such as: thefrugalshopper.com, simpleliving.net and frugaliving.com.

Learn to turn shopping time into activity time. Go for a bike ride, walk down memory lane, take the kids to the park; do anything and everything that you can to take your mind off shopping and spending. It works!

Step # 2: Time to Save!

There are any number of creative ways to live on less. However, you don't want to make your life miserable. Here are some great ways to economize without missing quality of life.

Don't think too much about it – just do it! Direct deposit is now your best friend! Your money is whisked away into your IRA, 401(k) or money market account—and you don't have to do a thing to make it happen. Just drop by your payroll department and/or your bank and fill out the forms. Do it today. Eat meatless some of the time. Go veggie. Prepare just three meatless days a week (without substituting pricey fish) and you could save $25 a week, which equals $100 a month, which equals $1,200 a year! Beans: You will learn to love them.

Play the money game. Whenever you get a $5 bill, put it aside for later. Alternatively, do the same with ones, with quarters or even all your spare change. You'll have a nest egg built up before you even miss a nickel. Never spend the extras. Save all of your income-tax refund, your holiday money from the folks, the $20.38 overpayment check from the telephone company and any other extras and save every penny.

Negotiate and Haggle. You will be impressed by who will drop their prices, fees and interest rates: airlines, hotels, credit card companies, and even computer/appliance/rug salespeople. Before you even think about paying full price: Haggle a bit first.

Re-evaluate your money before you spend. That dinner out for the family will cost more than you spend on groceries in a week. That fancy pair of shoes is worth half the cost of a commuter pass. Learn what your money is worth to you, and you won't be so quick to dispose of it.

Don't overpay on your taxes. Yes, you love to get a big refund from the IRS every spring. The fact is, though, you're effectively lending money to the government and interest-free. Go through your tax return and see if you can hold out until Dec. 31 to maybe get a $150 refund. That way you can use your money NOW should you need it for an emergency and bank the refund when you get it later.

Decide to raise your insurance deductibles. Reassess each of the deductibles for your various kinds of insurance. If you can raise them at all, your premiums will drop.

Bring your mortgage costs down. Look at whether or not the rate is too high. If it is, look to refinancing - this will save you money. Now, let's look at the private mortgage insurance (PMI) you've been paying because you didn't have enough money to make a 20% down payment. If the equity in your home is greater than 22%, make sure that it is cancelled. It's the law. Finally, pay up on your mortgage. If you can manage an extra $100 per month, you will save thousands in interest costs over the long haul.

Toss out those nasty, glossy catalogs. The best-known form of spending temptation known to man or woman is the catalogs. Sure they are fun and look good, but are they worth the risk of spending? Chuck them straight out into the trash.

Refuse those unnecessary fees. Like the $2.50 you pay just because the ATM is right there, right now as opposed to walking two blocks to your bank, where you don't get charged at all every time you use your cash card.

Alternatively, how about the late fees for returning videos? These really add up. Don't forget those fat charges banks hit you with when you write a check that, well, bounces.

Clean it yourself. I've discovered a very cool trick: When a clothing label says, "Dry Clean Only," I wash it. On the other hand, dab out that little mustard stain with an old-fashioned cleaning device cleverly known as a sponge.

Don't pay for a pro. If you can fix the neighbor's garage door and she can paint the kitchen: go for it and save.

Put your raise in the bank. Put that tiny 3% to 5% boost in the paycheck on your direct deposit and live on your previous salary.

Pay smart for long-distance. Evaluate all of the different telephone plans for value. Pay attention to what you are currently paying per minute. Some dial-around codes or cheap calling cards (one without a surcharge per call) may give you a better rate. Not only will you save, but also you may find you won't need to speak to Alvin in Schenectady so often.

Just buy the basics for the pets. Say no to pet pampering. Does your dog need those t-bone snacks? Does your cat need that rabbit-fur-lined toy? Probably not.

Vow never again to pay full price. The next time you must shop, hop onto the World Wide Web. Look for eBay, half.com and craigslist.org for excellent sources of "lightly used" goods—everything from books to jewelry to office furniture—even the entire first season of Star Trek on video.

When you are focused on being savings minded, you're thinking about money changes. Before you know it, you have substantial savings.

Smart Tips for Living on a Budget

Regardless of the time in history and no matter what the current state of the economy, no matter what the current trends are, no matter what the unemployment rate is or where interest rates are, some money-saving ideas always work and stay true.

Big changes come from small steps and if you determine to put even one of these many savings secrets into place, you will see big change in your life. You will now learn a variety of savings tips. You will learn how to best place your hard-earned money in a variety of down-to-earth ways. What you will learn about will set you up nicely in your day to day life.

Money Saving Tip #1:

The great Albert Einstein once said, "It takes a genius to see the obvious."

Let these wise words guide you today. What he meant by that is that sometimes the simpler things in life are the most powerful ... but because they are so obvious, we tend to ignore them, and not let them work for us.

One of the most powerful money making ideas is this: keep a daily diary of everything you spend. Go to the dollar store, buy a little book, and carry it with you wherever you go. Write down every penny – each single penny - you spend. It's just as simple as that.

If you do this one thing, you will find that something magical happens in your financial life in only a few weeks.

There is something incredibly powerful about writing down each of your expenditures. It makes the flow of money through your life more realistic and exacting. It shows you simply and clearly just exactly where you are spending your money, on what and why. Once you know this, it becomes much easier to control your spending. You will feel empowered with self-control and this will encourage saving.

Many people who have taken up this practice have not only learned something about themselves, which they never before understood, but they are often astounded by the simplicity of the lesson learned.

For example, a person could realize through examining their notebook that they actually spent nearly $1,000 throughout the year on diet soft drinks, snacks and candy bars! Since their job only brings in $20,000 per year, they realized that 5% of their entire income was being frittered away on something entirely frivolous. The person gave up the snacks and drinks, and found they had enough money to go on vacation the following year. If you had the choice between snacks and a much-needed vacation, which would you choose? Of course you would choose the vacation, we all would.

The point is, it was their daily expense log that helped achieve the insight and clarity they needed to realize control of their finances. That's what a simple spending record will do for you - it will give you much needed control over your spending, and thus your financial life. There may be nothing but a 75-cent notebook and a ballpoint pen between your life of financial struggle and financial freedom.

Money Saving Tip #2:

Stop deficit spending! We all know how Uncle Sam has been creating debt—spending more money than our country takes in. It's called deficit spending. Well, don't do the same! The same rules apply to you and me. Using those nasty little plastic cards may be the "American Way," but it's a debt making way and creates plenty of fools each new day.

Today, the average credit card holder is carrying around $8,000 in plastic debt!

Spending yourself into such debt with a credit card is certainly very easy, as many of you already know. The reason is psychological. When you give that clerk a credit card, it's just not the same as handing over a stack of green dollar bills. Would you as readily hand over a pocketful of ten-dollar bills as toss a credit card across a counter? Probably not. This one is a no-brainer for most!

Credit cards put you in debt and keep you there. Even for people with good incomes, paying your credit card debt down to zero can be amazingly difficult. In addition, make no bones about it; credit card debt will sap your financial strength just as readily as an open vein will deplete your physical body of its very life force. Using a credit card by choice can quickly turn to using it for need. Once you get to that point, you are already in trouble and it becomes time to get some help.

There is no secret in freeing yourself from the credit card game. You must take out a pair of scissors today, cut your cards in half, and begin paying them back, slowly but surely. Be sure to always pay more than the minimum amount due, even if it is only $10 more.

Once you stop adding to the debt, even small payments will eventually, add up. You can get out of debt, if you are patient and self-disciplined. Once your cards are history, you must adopt a strict pay-as-you go policy. Instead of buying now and paying later, save now and buy when you have the full amount. This is key to being able to save.

Once again, stopping credit-oriented consuming is one of the most powerful financial tools available to anyone today. Why not pick up this tool and use it for yourself?

Money Saving Tip #3:

Sell all of your junk. That's right; it's high past time for a serious yard sale. Search throughout your house or apartment for every single item that you don't really need, and then sell it all! Every last piece!

Take an inventory. The truth is, most people are astounded by what they own - and how much money they have tied up in items they no longer need and use. Why let it just sit and collect dust while it could collect interest instead in a savings account?

You could easily be $600, $1,200 ... even $5,000 richer by the end of the week. As an added bonus, you'd have your place cleaned up, and you will have a fresh feeling of beginning all over again. A garage sale is an excellent way to start. Not only do you clean out your house, but also it often gives a psychological boost that helps people get control of their life and money.

Money Saving Tip #4:

Ben Franklin said long ago: "A penny saved is a penny earned." Yes, it's still true and still one of the most powerful moneymaking tips in all of history. Understood well within Franklin's famous statement is the difficulty of saving.

It's tough to save and much easier to spend! We all know that! That's why every penny saved truly is earned - because it takes so much effort to hold on to that cash! If you can do it, it will work magic in your life. Having a savings account will de-stress your life. Imagine being ahead of your bills, rather than behind. When you are ahead of your bills, you entire life comes under your own control. You sleep better at night. Your mind is freer to come up with new ways to make more money and save more. Saving is contagious - once you let it get started!

<u>Some Tips to help you save:</u>

1. Don't settle for interest checking. Have a separate savings account that can't be as easily accessed as a checking account.

2. Keep your savings in a different bank - one that's off your regular route, or perhaps even in different town. That way you won't be tempted to dip into it every time you visit the bank to make a checking deposit.

3. Buy short-term savings bonds, which have 6-month to one-year maturity dates. You will get a higher rate, while at the same time keeping your money close in case of real money emergencies.

4. If you can, open the account under two, different names and require that both signatures be required to make a withdrawal. Two people can debate each withdrawal and keep each other in line.

5. When you get your paycheck, immediately put a minimum of 5% in your savings account. After just a year, you'll be amazed by how much you have actually saved and you will feel great about it.

Visualize abundance and wealth everyday. Am I actually suggesting that you practice some sort of mysticism that will make you into a "money magnet"? Perhaps yes, maybe no. Call it what you wish - a mind game, mysticism, New Age—the solid fact is that behind every wealthy man and woman is a positive attitude toward money.

Look at it like this: It costs ZERO one way or the other to have either negative or positive thoughts. So why not have positive thoughts AND increase the ODDS?

There have been many studies done on the thought patterns and the mind-set of some of the richest, most successful people in the world. The one thing that they all had in common was a positive attitude toward money and their ability to earn and keep it.

WHAT HAVE YOU LEARNED? RESPECT MONEY AND THINK POSITIVELY TOWARDS MONEY. THIS IS A GREAT START TO MEANINGFUL SAVINGS.

The key to being able to raise emergency money when needed most is to be in the right frame of mind about money in the first place. Think positive about money and spending and save. You can't beat that equation!

7 Serious Ways to Save Money – Not for the Faint of Heart

Do you truly want to save? Take a serious look at how you spend and then change it. Quit smoking those cigars, take in a roommate, park your car—and you'll save as much as $10,000 a year. It really is just as easy as all that!

Are you finding it harder and harder to blame savings shortfalls on your measly pay check?

Will it surprise you to learn that how much you save has little to do with your income? Well it is very true, in fact. It has more to do with whether you want to save and are willing to adjust your finances to boost your savings.

A recent study by Venti's and Wise, "Choice, Chance and Wealth Dispersion at Retirement," found a very wide range in how much people at the same income levels were able to save for retirement. The study pointed out that it wasn't just the higher income folks who managed to save the most. Indeed, even people in the lowest income groups were able to save more than some of their middle-income peers—by as much as $100,000.

What was their conclusion? Persons with little savings on the eve of retirement have simply chosen not to save as much and spend more over their lifetimes.

The key, then, is simple enough: Spend less than you earn and SAVE MORE. It is easy to see why some people get into financial trouble.

Some people don't stop and think that earning money is only one part of the financial health equation. The other critical part is learning how to manage money and save.

A big part of the problem for so many is that people just don't know enough about their own financial reality. They don't even know what they earn, they don't even know what it takes to live comfortably, and they don't even know their true, discretionary income."

What can be the solution?

People need to educate themselves. Sit down with your monthly bills and statements and figure out your real income and outgo. Then, decide if you like what you see. If not, create a realistic plan for changing it.

To help with the process, ask yourself these four essential questions:
What's my true and current financial picture?

- How do I choose to live?
- Can my current money support this and how do I really want to use my money?
- How can I best make use of my money?

Treat managing your money as if you would any other household chore and allot enough time for it each month.

Make note that: Many of the financial tools that have made life more convenient—such as credit cards—can promote very bad financial habits and prolong debt when misused. Credit cards should be used ONLY as the cash-management tool that they are and not as a borrowing tool.

Keep in mind that you are spending tomorrow's money when you put things on a credit card. You keep locking yourself up and losing your freedom, bit by bit.

The bottom line on financial health is Stop Spending

<u>More Serious Savings Strategies</u>

If you are serious about having a healthy emergency money fund, you might want to curb the consumer in you. This means, instead of spending, saving. Of course, the number one, best way of saving remains to have a portion of your weekly paycheck automatically deposited to your savings account. If you like the idea of deciding, week by week, how much savings you will deposit, take heart and adapt a serious tip or two. It's all good if the end result is better and more savings.

Hold that "mother" of all garage sales, once and for all! Do your homework and literally do a house inventory. Journey back, all the way back, into the furthest reach of every closet and decide that, if you have not used it for more than six months, it will have to go. Most people have at least $1,000 worth of garage sale items hidden away in their home. This turns out to be a veritable gold mine for many.

Just how much do you need that nasty, pack-a-day smoking habit? In Washington state, that's easily $5 a day—or about $1,800 a year—that can go right into your savings. This does not even begin to touch the savings in insurance and health care.

Tame the driving tiger in you. Instead, carpool or use public transportation. This will save you on gas, insurance and maintenance costs—not to mention any money spent on a headache. Using the IRS's 2002 mileage reimbursement rate of 36.5 cents per mile as a proxy for the cost of commuting, you could save $1,141 a year by driving half the time for 50 weeks of the year (based on a 25-mile roundtrip commute). For an even more serious approach, consider nixing your car if you live in the city. Some cities are now implementing progressive programs that allow you to have access to a car without the ownership hassles (e.g. "Flexcar" in Seattle, Portland and Washington, D.C.)

Buy items used. The average consumer spends about $1,750 a year on clothing and its upkeep, according to the U.S. Bureau of Labor Statistics' most recent Consumer Expenditure Survey. You can easily cut that in half by shopping at consignment shops and auctions, though the life of the goods may be a bit less than buying new. To account for that, the annual savings may only amount to 25%, or $437.

Become a homebody. At just over $1,800 a year on average, entertainment spending has a way of eating up the best-planned budgets. Consider the library for books, music and movies. Eat out less often. The average person spends $2,276 a year on eating out. Try cutting your spending in half on both areas for annual savings of more than $1,900.

Cut your housing costs. While a move across the tracks may save some money, moves are expensive. Consider renting out a room in your house. The average housing costs per person in 2004 were just over $13,200. In metropolitan areas such as Seattle, rooms easily go for $400 a month. Figure about $20 of that goes to increases in utility costs, and you've still realized annual savings of more than $4,000 before any income taxes.

Cut up every one of your credit cards. Build an emergency fund first to handle most unexpected expenses. This allows you to become your own lending agency. Credit cards can be a cash-flow management tool, but paying only the minimum will keep you in debt for years.

If you're the average American with at least one credit card, you probably have close to $8,523 in credit card debt, according to industry research group CardWeb.com. At an average APR of 14.4%, it could cost you as much as $1,100 a year in interest rates alone. By simply waiting until you've saved enough money to make purchases, you could eliminate those interest payments.

If you're very ambitious and follow all the above tips, you could be looking at savings of some $12,000 a year. Figuring you can invest that at the historical rate of return of 10%, your savings do start to compound nicely—and rapidly. Instead of the debt, go for the emergency fund and save.

Make Small Cuts for Huge Savings

Tilt the wheel of creating wealth in your favor. Naturally, spending less is one way. However, to be sure to make your money work harder for you—set goals to make certain it happens.

Many have wondered what can be the foolproof way of creating wealth. Is it to buy top paying Internet stocks or to work for a tech startup that offers you valuable stock options? Is the trick to count every penny or is the road to wealth paved with risk? Do you have to be especially smart and well-connected? Alternatively, is becoming wealthy a matter of luck?

The answer is: There is no one, true road to wealth, and all of the above have created wealth for more than just a few notable individuals. Nevertheless, you can put the odds of creating wealth on your side by following a few simple precepts.

1. Spend less than what you earn.

This can be the most overlooked scenario, because many people believe it's a matter of cutting back on your current standard of living—a strategy that's far too difficult for many people. Yes, you can affect your personal balance sheet by spending less money eating out or on entertaining out. Making a pot of coffee at the office instead of buying a $3 espresso will make a small difference in your cash flow. Nevertheless, the biggest difference will be made on the income side of the ledger.

If you wish to get on the right road to saving, stop looking at your budget as a pie that must be cut up into various size pieces. Instead, of trying to figure out how the different pieces will cover your expenses, concentrate on how you will expand the size of the pie. Yes, you could ask your boss for a raise. At the same time, figure out how you can begin to earn more money on the side. Start thinking about how you will sweeten the existing pie.

Think about how you're spending your time, as well as your money. Perhaps instead of taking the family out this weekend, you could earn an extra $80 by becoming a waiter or bartender. Instead of taking the kids shopping at the mall, you could work as a salesclerk earning some extra cash.

If you don't wish to work every weekend, think about working every other weekend to start. Instead of paying for a baby sitter while you attend a concert, take care of a few other children on Saturday or Sunday, freeing working parents to do their errands. When it comes your weekend to work, do a switch. This will save you time and money.

Then, instead of spending the extra money you earn from your part-time work, you can invest it so the money can work for you. When you do this, you will learn to appreciate your free time that much more.

2. Make your money work for you.

The ultimate secret to financial success lies in having your money do the work, so you can relax. This requires accumulating enough investment dollars so that the growth and earnings can free you from the need to work even harder. The last thing you will want to be doing is punching a time clock.

Plenty of very wealthy people continue on working simply because they enjoy what they're doing so much. They also redefine work to include managing their money. For the wealthy, the two can go hand in hand.

Every where you go you will hear, "I never get to the point where I won't have to return to work because I can't afford to set money aside today. These people overlook the power of compound interest.

Every worker with earned income is now entitled to open a non-deductible IRA or, even better, a Roth IRA. The maximum $3,000-a-year contribution works out to a cost of $57.69 a week. Any hard working American is capable of achieving this goal.

Moreover, a $3,000 annual investment in a Roth IRA, growing tax-free at the historical average of 10.6% for the stock market, builds to more than $500,000 in 30 years. If you start in your twenties and put $3,000 in that same Roth IRA every year, at 10.6%, you could have a nest egg of nearly, $5.2 million at age 70, according to the MSN Money's Savings Calculator. Even with an 8% annual return, you'll end up with $1.9 million.

3. Be sure your money is working for you, instead of against you.

Your money can work very powerfully for you if you make the right decisions and implement a plan of regular investing. At the same time, wrong money decisions will place deep potholes on your road to success.

The classic example is credit-card debt. Consider the example of a person who charges $2,000 on a credit card at 19.8% interest and a $40 annual fee. If you make only the minimum monthly payments (and many people do just that), it will take you 31 years and two months to pay off the balance! Moreover, along the way, you'll pay an additional $8,202 in finance charges. This is absurd logic!

What could possibly be so important to charge today that it puts you in debt for a period far longer than the object is likely to last? (Sure, a mortgage lasts 30 years, but the interest is deductible and your home should grow in value over that time.) Most things that you want to charge on your card have a far shorter life. For many, they can do entirely without that one purchase.

If you're already in debt, if you would only double the minimum monthly payment, you could be out of debt in less than three years. Paying down current debt is the smartest way to start on the road to financial freedom.

4. Keep a tight clasp on that wallet

When you take a close look at your paycheck, you'll notice many deductions before you get to the amount you can cash or put in the bank. Surely, there are deductions for Social Security, federal, and perhaps state income taxes.

It's money that's out of your paycheck before you have a chance to even make decisions about it. Money set aside for wealth building should be treated in the exact same way. If your company offers a 401(k) retirement plan, make sure you sign up for the maximum possible contribution. It will be taken out of your paycheck, each pay period, automatically. (And if your company matches all or part of your contribution, failing to sign up is like walking away from free money!)

If you didn't have a chance for automatic deductions to a company savings plan or even a U.S. Savings Bonds payroll deduction plan, then you'll have to create your own automatic savings plan. Ask if your company will deposit your paycheck directly into your bank account—or promise yourself to do it the day you receive the check.

Then sign up for an automatic monthly deduction plan with a mutual fund company to create regular deposits into an IRA. You can even set up an automatic deduction for U.S. Savings bonds at its Web site. The whole point to this is to get the money out of your checking account as quickly as possible, before you see it and spend it.

5. Create money savings and investment goals.

Would you like to have $1 million by the age of 40 or 50 or by the time you retire? Sure you would!

Begin by setting your own goals. Never set a goal you can't control. Your targets can't depend on your boss giving you a raise; they must be reachable by your own efforts. You might need to invest in yourself by acquiring more education or training so you can qualify for a job that pays more.

You might need to take more risk in your investments or in your lifestyle by taking on a second job that pays commissions instead of a fixed salary. Evaluate the risks involved, and understand that by putting the odds on your side, you can get a larger return.

Emergency Money Strategy while Dealing With Debt, Financial Stress & Family

Financial stress is common among those forced into frugality because of a lost job, divorce, death in the family, or being overcome with debt, etc. This can cause a person to feel insecure, fearful, anxious, angry, and, of course, depressed.

These same feelings are easily the number one cause of poor money management decisions. These poor decisions will lead to unmanageable debt loads, and start a vicious cycle of panic that never seems to end.

When you reach this point, and you find yourself with a money emergency, your feelings of helplessness can become so overwhelming you literally stop functioning in the real world.

YOU NEED TO HAVE YOUR WITS ABOUT YOU TO RAISE EMERGENCY MONEY

Get yourself Immediate Help

If you recognize any of the above traits in yourself, get the help you need right away. See out a professional counselor ... talk to a friend or family member ... but talk to someone! If you know someone who is exhibiting the above traits, offer to help them! It doesn't matter whether you lend then cash, an ear, offer some helpful advice, or help them get counseling, do something!

The first thing that you need to grasp is that no situation is hopeless. With just a little guidance and patience, along with a couple of well thought out goals, and emotional support from family and friends, you can do what it takes to come out of dire circumstances.

You can adapt a new outlook, new skills, and best of all, a new feeling of self-esteem. Don't allow anyone to tell you different, and if they do, close the same door that they came into and don't again open it! What you need is positive reinforcement and not negativity to help you get to the other side.

Seek out your True Friends

When you are desperate to raise emergency funds, it usually doesn't take very long for you to realize who really cares about you, who is truly a friend ... be they family or not. Your friends will be there for you in your time of need, offer encouragement, and lend an ear so you can just talk. Ask for help in coming up with good ideas about how you can raise emergency funds during such a difficult time in your life. Be open to the many suggestions that you will receive.

Prepare to Set your Priorities

There comes the time when you will need to put aside your feelings and just concentrate on the well being of you, and your family. This has to be your priority during times of financial stress and upheaval. In financially stressful times, if you, as the Mom or Dad, can't cope, how can you expect your children to cope now, or in the future? You must set the example for the rest of the family to draw strength from them.

So make the decision today to learn how to cope, to make the changes you can, to stay focused and goal-oriented, and to let anxiety and financial stress go out the door so that you will be prepared to deal with any money emergencies that come your way.

You need to be able to come up with some quick cash fixes (without additional borrowing) to recover from a Money Emergency:

Budgeting Tip #1: The first thing you want to do is prioritize to get back on track very quickly. If that means letting your credit card bill go for a bit, so be it. As soon as you realize that you have a money emergency, contact your credit card issuers and request reduced interest rates and payments. Not only one, both!

Budgeting Tip #2: For your car payment, call the creditor and request a payment extension. Perhaps you hate payment extensions, because they require a fee and you still have to make the payment at the end of the contract. In this case, a payment extension can allow a little breathing room to help you recover during your money emergency. Expect that you will likely have to pay a fee (usually about ¼ - 1/3 the car payment amount) for the extension. Freeing up the money you need today is your first and only goal at this point.

Budgeting Tip #3: Check to see if your mortgage holder will allow an extension for a nominal fee. Do this today!

Budgeting Tip #4: Another quick fix, is to host an on the spot yard sale. You don't have too much time for planning, so do a quick survey of your personal belongings. Come up with clothes that no longer fit, but that are in good condition, knick-knacks, dishes, and books as well as stuff you bought but no longer use. Throw it all together, quickly. Put some notices up the same day at laundry mats and grocery stores around town, and remember to place a sign at the end of your driveway. You can make a quick $300 this way with very little time and effort.

Budgeting Tip #5: If you have a larger item to sell, call into the local radio stations to see if they have a "call in swap show" on the weekends. This is a very popular way to quickly convert gently used and more expensive items to fast cash.

Budgeting Tip #6: Another quick option is with utility and telephone bills. If you aren't already on a budget plan, ask that the current bill (plus any previous balance you owe) be set up for a budget plan. Expect to pay a down payment (usually ¼ of the bill) and that all future bills (while on the back payment budget plan) must be kept current. The nice thing about it ... it's usually interest free, and can give you some much-needed breathing space for a month. You must be sure though that you maintain the regular utility payments AND the budget payments in the coming month.

Budgeting Tip #7: Check with your family church regarding emergency help. Local churches can be one of the best places to find out what's available in the community to help those in need, or in times of emergency. Check with your local church, first.

Getting Fast Cash through Borrowing

If you are absolutely, positively, in a bind, a real cash emergency, and you have exhausted all of the above, then consider borrowing. First, ask your family, then your local bank.

As a last resort, you may want to consider what's known as a "Payday Loan." These types of borrowing stores can be useful when all else fails.

A Few Timely Lessons in Simple Living

Planning for a money emergency takes plenty of forethought. It is best to start to plan now rather than need to scramble to come up with the cash when the need is greatest.

- Adapt some strategic thinking.

- Reprogram your mind now to become a saver

- Simple living yields simply millions in savings
- Remind yourself that you can do with less

- Make a mindful decision to live light.
- Put your entire family on a budget

- Discuss strategies about how to build your first budget

Better Money Management Thinking

The first step to making better choices when it comes to how we spend our money or time is living and acting consciously and examining daily money and work habits.

Simple living is largely a matter of making better choices in life: about how we spend, consume, create community and spend our free time.

It is NOT to just consume less. It is to consume smarter OR differently. We must NOT just go blindly along when it comes to consumption.

Just say no to impulse buying

- If you see something you want, put it aside and think about it for at least a couple of days. Chances are, the impulse should pass.
- Look to other sources of entertainment

- Find ways to socialize and create your own entertainment that don't revolve around expensive restaurant tabs or event tickets.
- Spend time in quiet time

- Quiet time helps you recharge your spiritual batteries and give you the time you need to reflect on life and make better choices.

- Remember that time is money after all

- This time issue is going to loom even larger than money. We, as a society, have concluded that time is money. The two are closely tied. Spend time wisely.

Every Day Money Saving Tips

How to Save Money on Gas

Gas prices just keep going up, and our wallets keep decreasing in size. This how-to will teach you many ways to save money at the local gas station.

Steps

1. Take out a credit card. Some credit cards offer gas savings when you use the card for purchases. This works in much the same way that some credit card companies give you frequent flyer miles when you use their card for purchases.

2. Get a gas membership card. Look for membership benefits. In addition, department and grocery stores give discounts at the fuel pump when you use their store membership cards. Shopping at Giant Eagle grocery store and using their membership card, it's possible (at the time of this writing) to fill a car's tank for .79 cents a gallon, with savings of $1.36 per gallon.

3. Give your car a good tune up. While giving your car a tune up won't actually save you money at the pump, it will save you in gas. Using less gas saves you money over all. Have the oil changed, and have a certified mechanic give your engine a twice over.

4. Check the WWW for deals. Web sites let you find the best deals in your area.

5. Buy a hybrid car. Not only do hybrid cars give you immediate savings at the pump, the U.S. government and your local state offer tax breaks for people that use gas saving cars. Federal deductions for using gas saving cars can be as high as $2000. If you can't afford the growing number of hybrid cars out there, consider getting a regular car with good MPG (miles per gallon), like the Toyota Echo.

6. Turn off the AC. Running the car's air conditioning puts extra strain on your car's engine. This translates into you car eating up more gas per mile. Use less gas, save money. Depending on the car you drive, at highway speeds, the AC might put less drag on your car than if all the windows are open. Therefore, you might want to keep it cool on the highway.

7. Use the cheaper stuff. Most modern cars run just as well with the cheap gas as they do with the more expensive gas. In fact, engineers assume the car buyer is going to use the cheap gas, and so, they design the car's engine accordingly.

8. Don't fill the tank when prices are higher. Gas suppliers and gas station owners can charge high prices for gas because they know people will pay for it. The owners monitor how much gas people are putting into their cars each day. If they hike up the price a few cents and people are still filling up their tanks, this tells the owners that people are willing to pay the high price. Adding only a few gallons to your car when prices are high sends a message to the owners that people are not happy about the high prices.

9. Don't drive. Don't drive when you don't absolutely have to. Carpooling, walking, taking the bus, and riding a bike not only saves you gas, but these are better for the environment and may be better for your health. Do you really need to drive to the store when it is only a couple of blocks down the street?

10. Check the tire air pressures weekly. Buy an inexpensive manual air pump and an accurate tire gauge (not a pencil gauge as they are not accurate). Keep all tires inflated to the same pressure as recommended for your car but not for your tire. Go by the sticker on the doorframe and not the tire wall.

11. Drive at a consistent speed and keep the windows up tight. Keeping the windows closed reduces the drag on your car. Sticking to the speed limit also helps. So, will using less gear changes and revving the engine less. Avoid accelerating fast or braking suddenly. Use cruise control when you can.

12. Clean out any unnecessary items in your car. If you have heavy objects in your car that you don't need - remove them. If your car is lighter, it will use less fuel to get you to where you're going.

13. Avoid leaving your car idle. If you are going to be stopped for more than one minute, you will save gas by turning the car off and restarting when you are ready to go.

14. Buy on cold days. Buy fuel on cold days and if you can, drive on the hot days. When you buy on cold days, and pay for volume, you buy more "mass" of fuel for the same price. Never fill the tank completely or it will overflow when it becomes hotter.

Simpler Solutions for Managing your Money

Let's face it, coming up with smart and simple ways of saving money takes thinking that is a bit more creative.

Use some of these shortcuts to managing your finances. They are guaranteed to save you time and money.

Trick your mind into saving
Can't always come up with where your money goes? There is a simple solution: Trick your own mind into spending less and saving more.

If you are up for a challenge, allocate yourself a weekly allowance. Put a set amount of allowance into an envelope and determine that this will be all you will be allowed to spend for any given week. Next, divide your allowance to take care of your expenses. When you get down to the last $20, that's the amount you put into your emergency fund. When the money is gone, there will be no more until next week.

Each payday, allocate a percentage to go into a secret fund used only for emergencies. When it's crunch time, you will know it's there.

Establish one dresser drawer just to toss single dollar bills. This way when the pizza man arrives, you will have the singles handy and won't need to break the larger dollar amounts. This discipline forces your mind to think larger amounts and to save larger amounts. You get into the habit of spending only the singles. This works!

To control your credit card debt, carry just one card and pay it off each month. If you are tempted to over spend, the credit card goes into the safe where you only stash your emergency fund. When crunch day comes you have a credit card you can use that will always be in good standing.

Jot down expenses in a notebook and tally them at the end of each week to see if you are over or under your budget estimates. Build in more than you need so that you will always have a cushion in case of a cash emergency. Tracking your spending takes some work but if you take careful notes, you will always be able to see one or two areas where you're leaking cash. You can then come up with an extra $20 or more per week in savings. That's $1,000 a year in real money for an emergency fund.

More tricks to add to your own savings routine:
Have your paycheck automatically deposited directly to savings rather than to your checking account. You will transfer money to pay your bills, but you'll think twice about withdrawing additional cash.

Make ONLY one ATM withdrawal each week.
Subtract your credit card purchases immediately from your checking account so you're not surprised once the bill arrives.

When you pay off a loan, add the amount to payments you're already making to the next lender on your list. You can also send the money to a saving or investment account earmarked for a house, a vacation or a new car and this money will be made available in case of a money emergency.

PAY YOUR BILLS ONLINE AND SAVE

Nearly one-third of U.S. consumers pay their bills online, says Judy Wicks of CheckFree, the leading provider of electronic-billing and payment services. Probably the easiest way to pay your bills online is to use a safe, encrypted service—offered by banks, credit unions, brokers and companies such as AOL, MSN, Quicken or Yahoo! Arrange for an e-mail reminder that a bill is due.

The service can handle payments entirely electronically or it can generate a paper check, if necessary—to pay the guy who mows your lawn, for example. If a payment is late, many bill-paying services will reimburse you for late fees up to a certain amount (sometimes as much as $50), as long as you have scheduled the payment within their guidelines.

To shed yet more paperwork, arrange to receive bills and statements electronically. Sign up with e-billers on many services or at MyCheckFree.com.

Online bill paying also helps you to keep your finances organized. You have your records right there—what you owe, past payments—and all on one site.

Wells Fargo goes a step further: Its online-banking customers have access to My Spending Report, which they can use as a de facto budget. My Spending Report tracks online bill payments and Wells Fargo debit- and credit-card charges, and plugs them into one of 20 categories so that you can see how much you've spent on, say, movies and restaurant meals.

In addition, of course, you can track your spending using Microsoft Money or Quicken. With Quicken 2006, once you pay a bill there's no need to print and file it. Instead, you can attach the bill electronically to the account from which you made your payment, so it's always at your fingertips.

REWARD YOURSELF

Are you trying to figure out which credit card offers the best rebate? Simple solution: Take the cash and run.

It couldn't be easier than this. With a cash rebate, you get either a check in the mail or a credit on your statement, so you don't have to weigh the relative benefits of airline miles versus a new set of luggage. To find the best deals, we simplified the process by assuming that you spend $33 on gas each week, $100 a week on groceries and $1,000 per month on other purchases.

Tops is the Citi Dividend Platinum Select card (at . It charges 11.74% and offers rebates of 5% on purchases at supermarkets, drugstores and gas stations and 1% on everything else. However, Citi caps its annual rebate at $300, which you would reach in about eight months under our scenario (at that point you could switch to another card). Exempt from the cap are goods bought through Citi's Dividend Merchant Network, which includes more than 200 retailers, catalogs and Internet sites. Those purchases earn rebates between 5% and 7%.

Next up is the National City Everyday Rewards Elite Visa card (at , on which our yearlong spending spree would earn a rebate of $270. National City is unique in bundling restaurants with grocery stores in a single category, with rebates of 2%. With an interest rate of 10.49%, the card rebates 4% on gas, 3% on movies and up to 1% on everything else. There are spending caps in some categories.

The American Express Blue Cash card (at www.americanexpress.com) carries an interest rate of 11.24%. It gives you up to 5% on groceries, gas and drugstore purchases, and up to 1.5% on the rest of your charges, up to a maximum expenditure of $50,000. Total rebate in our example: $266.

The Capital One No Hassle Cash card (at www.capitalone.com) offers a rebate of up to 3% on gas and groceries and 1% on everything else you buy, with no dollar limit and a relatively modest 9.9% interest rate. You would earn an annual reward of $237 in our scenario.

The Chase Free Cash Rewards Platinum Visa card (at , which carries an interest rate of 11.99%, gives you one point for every dollar spent on purchases (with a $60,000 spending cap). In addition, it has an interesting twist: a one-point bonus for every dollar you pay in interest. Each time you accrue 2,500 points, you receive a check for $25. Without the interest bonus, you'd be eligible for a rebate of $189, so the card is more attractive for card users who often carry a balance.

When saving for an emergency fund – you just can't go wrong with cash!

Multiple Ways to make the most of a Year-end Bonus

If you have a nice chunk of extra cash to look forward to each year, think now about the best ways to put it to work for you.

Maybe this year you'll get lucky. You've applied for that great, higher-paying promotion and this will boost your monthly pay by $500. You want to make sure the money goes toward building a better future rather than being squandered on items, you just don't need.

That's the beauty of getting a year-end raise or bonus—it's one of the rare opportunities to make a big difference in your finances without having to make sacrifices. You've been living without the money previously, so you can take any financial medicine you need even without altering your present lifestyle.

Financial triage

Consider first that all extra cash should first be used to solidify your base. Next, pay off all credit-card debt.

This can have a gigantic ripple effect on the rest of your finances. As soon as you stop paying higher interest charges each month, you'll have more money to devote to any other goals.

Pad your emergency fund, if you don't already have three to six months' worth of living expenses in a safe and liquid account. That way you won't have to go into debt or raid long-term savings for unexpected bills when the bigger emergencies do arrive.

Add contributions to your 401(k), if you haven't hit the limit. You'll avoid paying more taxes on the extra cash, and you may earn free money if you get an employer match. You can also invest part of your bonus in your IRA if you haven't contributed $3,000 for 2004 ($3,500 if you're 50 or older). If you've already reached that limit, use your bonus to make your 2005 IRA contribution in January (the limit rises to $4,000 next year, $4,500 if you're 50 or older) or earmark a bigger chunk of your raise each month.

Take a look at that long-term debt

Now that you have boosted your financial foundation, you have more flexibility. Watson is already in great shape—she's maxing out her 401(k) and Roth IRA contributions—but she still has about $17,000 in student loans hanging over her head. The loans carry a low, 3.5% rate, so she's trying to choose between adding the $500 a month to her loan payments or investing the extra money.

With interest rates that low, paying off the loan doesn't need to be a priority. "If you can earn at least 3.5% in the marketplace, and I believe that you can, then *investing is the better way to go*," says Brian Jones, a certified financial planner in Fairfax, Va. Investing becomes even more important if you need to save for a short-term goal, such as buying a house.

However, it's okay if you'd rather pay off a student loan to get it out of the way. "Psychologically, it's important to get these debts behind you before you start to move ahead," says Mari Adam, a certified financial planner in Boca Raton, Fla. "I know people in their 30's who still have big loans, and that debt becomes like a ball and chain around their leg."

The same is true if you're thinking of devoting part of your raise to making extra mortgage payments. Chris Crocket, a doctor in Tupelo, Miss., is getting a big bonus this year that could be enough to pay off his mortgage that has 10 years remaining at 4.75%. As long as he's covered his other bases, paying off the loan could give him the equivalent of a guaranteed 4.75% return.

Eliminating your mortgage payment can also help if you'll be retiring soon or worry that you may lose your job, says Evelyn D'Amico, a financial planner in Paoli, Pa. However, you don't want to tie up too much money in a single investment. For better diversification, you could devote part of your raise or bonus to your mortgage and then invest the rest.

Don't forget to treat yourself
It is time to have some fun and you deserve it! You worked hard for your bonus or raise, so, go out there and have some fun.
You can set up a vacation fund.

Use part of your extra cash today to pay for the trip you have always wanted. You only need to set aside $310 per month in a savings account paying 2% to end up with $5,000 for springtime in Italy in 2006. Imagine spending the spring in Italy! Now that would be some kind of vacation.

Spend some money on your home.
Many home improvements can save you big money over the long haul. For example, think about the value of storm-resistant windows and shutters. Spending an extra few thousand dollars now, not only helps protects your home, but also can increase its value and lower the premiums on your homeowner's policy. This is smart planning!

One final idea is to start up a charitable fund. With $10,000, you can set up a donor-advised fund at many mutual fund companies and brokerage firms. You can then deduct the contributions on your tax return straight away and decide later which charities that you wish to support.

A Few Useful Savings Strategies

1. Don't pay a dime for anything that you can make or fix for yourself.

2. Prolong the life of whatever you own.

3. Use less of what you need.

4. Think creatively. The answer doesn't have to be "buy a new one."

5. Don't toss anything if it can be reused or recycled somehow.

You could do these tried-and-true, pioneer values now.

If you really want to save money, you can't just look at ways to save now. You have to look at your life, today.

Simple Ways to Bring both Calm AND Savings into your Life

Saving is far more than just an action – it is a way of living, day-by-day.

—

Start to be calm by first slowing. Whatever it is that you are working on now, stop. Spend the next 30 minutes a day in silence and solitude. You need to teach your mind how to relax, so you can shift from the work-and-spend treadmill and then focus on what's most important to you.

A calm heart is a tidy heart. It is time to clean up your act. Start today by spending 15 minutes every day going through a closet, a shelf, a drawer, and getting rid of anything you don't use or cherish. Once you start on these surface areas, weeding that out, the skills and mindset carry over to more complex areas like your work, money and relationships.

It is now time to learn what is enough. Being calm and saving is really about transforming your life in a conscious and deliberate manner. It is determining what is enough in your life, so that you can do more with even less.
Finally, seek out some good support—whether you're trying to save money or simplify your life.

Don't go this alone. With Americans $2 trillion deep in debt, you're certainly not alone in your desire to save money. Find a friend who can help you to get started and then get busy. You will be glad that you did.

Slash your electric bill in 6 easy steps

Spending lots to save pennies makes very little sense, but if you're already in the market for a new appliance, consider the Web as your first line of defense in energy-savings.

Perhaps you weren't so Eco-conscious until that glaring electric bill landed in your mailbox. It's time to become mindful of the green in your wallet and save energy at the same time.

Start by simply unplugging unused appliances, lowering the temperature on your electric water heater to 120 degrees F, and washing only full loads of dishes and air drying them.

At the same time take a look at the free online calculators to get customized tips for improving your home's energy efficiency at Home Energy Saver, a Web site sponsored by the U.S. Environmental Protection Agency (EPA) and the Department of Energy (DOE).

Spending hundreds to save pennies generally doesn't make sense, but if you're already in the market for a new appliance, or even light bulbs, consider the Web your first energy-savings tool.

Think Climate Control
A typical household uses the bulk of its energy for heating and cooling—up to 44% of your utility bill, according to the DOE's Energy Efficiency and Renewable Energy Network (EREN).

Install a programmable thermostat. This can reduce energy wasted while heating or cooling a house when no one is home or everyone's asleep.

According to the Home Energy Saver site, Energy Star programmable thermostats can save as much as 20% to 30% on your heating or cooling costs by allowing for multiple daily settings and automatically adjusting when the outside temperature changes. Participating manufacturers include Honeywell, Hunter Fan and Smart Systems International. Unfortunately, it's not easy to search for programmable thermostats by Energy Star status. Instead, keep an eye out for those with features typical of the Energy Star thermostats: temperature recovery systems, two programs and four temperature settings.

Think Ceiling fans
When you move the air, you tend to feel cooler. This allows for higher summertime thermostat settings. According to EREN, the effect is equivalent to lowering the air temperature by about 4° F (2° C), and using less energy than air conditioners in doing so.

Think Lighting, Cooking and other Appliances
The next-biggest household energy use after climate control is for lighting, cooking and other appliances. Not counting the fridge, these make up about 33% of a typical utility bill.

Think Compact Fluorescent Lamps (CFL's)
CFL's will use up to 75% less energy than standard incandescent bulbs and will last up to 10 times longer, according to Home Energy Saver. This is very good, because they're also more expensive to start with.

Check your local utility for ideas. Look for a free "Conservation Kit", containing among other things, two CFL's. This, of course, is a terrific deal!

Think Energy-efficient Appliances
Use the Energy Star site as a starting point to search for Maytag washing machines. Look for the Atlantis MAV9600 high-efficiency model for $689 at

Best Maytag.

Among household appliances, the refrigerator is likely your biggest energy consumer, especially if it's more than 15 years old. It can account for up to 9% of your energy costs alone. Again, look to the Energy Star site for a list of energy-efficient models if you're looking to replace yours.

Hot Water Heating
Heating water is the third-biggest home-energy cost and typically accounts for 14%-20% of your total energy bill.

Think Hot Water Jackets
Hot water jackets usually sell for $10 to $20, and shipping charges for buying them online can easily increase their cost by 50% or more. Use the Web to find offline deals in this case.

Think Aerating, Low-flow Faucets and Showerheads
Both Niagara and AM Conservation models popped up on a variety of environmental sites, including EnergyGuide, which also had the best price for the four-way adjustable Niagara showerhead at $6.75. The nice thing about ordering from EnergyGuide is that it automatically searches for any rebates based on the ZIP code you enter.

When you're considering buying a new home, you can plan for energy savings from the ground up with an energy-efficient homebuilding project. Check the DOE's Building America and the EPA sites to find projects near you.

GOOD WAYS TO FIND FREE MONEY

If you are tired of making lifestyle changes to accommodate your savings plans then read on. These ideas lead you to prime places to look for money that's already rightfully yours.

Some people see little point in changing their ways to save a quick $5 or $10. These same people find it difficult to believe such small amounts can actually make a significant difference to their bottom line. They'd much rather indulge in a little daily luxury, like enjoying a cup of espresso each day, then tighten their belts for what they see as measly savings.

For all the spendthrifts at heart, here are some concrete ways to save on things you are already paying for. No need to change your lifestyle or habits in the least. Think of it as money that you are already overpaying to others.

Step up to the plate and claim your free money!

Talking on your cell-phone
You thought you were going to need 2,000 minutes a month, only to find 300 or even 200 would do just as well.

If you're coming to the end of your contract, or if your service provider is willing to waive the early-termination fee, ask to have your deal changed as soon as possible.

Think about this: Verizon's America's Choice 3,200-minute plan runs about $200 per month; you'll spend just $40 for its 400-minute America's Choice plan. This is provided you don't start going over on your minutes and incurring pricey overage charges, that's $160 in savings each month, or $1,920 a year. Even changing from the America's Choice 1,100-minute plan at $80, would still cut your telephone bill in half for an added $480 in your pocket.

Local and long-distance calling: If you're not using all of your cell-phone minutes each month on a plan that doesn't allow you to just roll them over, you can at least offset your landline costs with those otherwise-wasted minutes. Are you already doing this? Try bundling your local and long-distance plans if you're regularly spending more than $50 per month. Many bundled plans start at just $50 before taxes and fees and allow you to talk for as long as you want without the huge bills.

Calculate all of the above carefully, though. If your usage is not steady, you'll pay the same rate every month, meaning no breaks for vacations when your usage normally decreases.

Your checking account: When was the last time you looked at the monthly fees your bank assesses on your checking account? By switching to a non-interest-bearing account, you can pay far less money and avoid higher fees.

Bankrate.com's annual survey of checking accounts found that average monthly fees are up to $10.86 on interest-bearing accounts, vs. $3.72 for regular checking accounts. You'll have to keep $2,258 socked away in that interest-bearing account to avoid fees versus the $245 minimum for the non-interest account. So, what are you giving up?

Average yields sat at a paltry 0.27% in the fall of 2003, the time of the Bankrate report. Meantime, if you can, try to plan your ATM withdrawals. The average fee you'll pay for using another bank's ATM machine is $2.69 -- $1.40 to the ATM's bank and $1.29 to your own. Eliminating only one of these withdrawals each week can save you a nice $140 per year.

Your insurance: You can save on your insurance policies in a variety of ways. Ask your insurance provider outright for discounts: Besides the usual good student and safety discounts on auto policies, ask for a multi-policy discounts if you're insuring more than one vehicle. Raise your deductibles on older cars or drop collision coverage altogether if your car is worth less than $1,000. Raising your deductible from $200 to $500 can reduce your premium by as much as 30%, according to Insure.com.

NEVER overpay to borrow your credit cards. Do you think that 2% or 3% isn't worth fighting for on your credit card's APR? Consider this: If you're an average American, you owe $8,940 in household credit card debt, according to CardWeb.com's CardData Service. At the average APR of 16.44%, you'll pay $1,470 per year just in interest alone.

For every 1% decrease in APR, you will save $89. However, the difference is far more dramatic over the entire life of your debt. Figuring you can make monthly payments of 5% of your debt per month, you'll pay $3,334 in total interest at the higher rate. However, at an APR of 13.44%, you'll have paid $2,551 - that is 23% less.

Also, lots of cards come with added benefits, such as airline miles or, better yet, even cash back. American Express' Blue Cash card rewards you with up to 5% cash back; the GM card awards 5% back toward a GM new car purchase or lease. On the average credit card debt of $8,940, that works out to $447. Use MSN Money's Credit Card Analyzer to find other low-rate and cash-back cards. In addition, you can check CardWeb for a list of the monthly rewards that credit cards are offering.

Your mortgage. Your biggest savings potential here is to get rid of PMI, or private mortgage insurance. PMI protects the lender should you default on your loan. You're obligated to pay this so long as your equity remains below 20%, but once you cross that magic threshold, you should ask your lender to drop the fee.

The law actually says your lender must drop the fee once your equity crosses 22%, provided you have a conventional loan originated or refinanced after July 29, 1999 and you have a good payment history. However, if you have an older loan, you could be paying this unnecessarily without realizing it.

Depending on the size of your mortgage, this could be adding hundreds of dollars to your mortgage cost annually. Look into this, today.

Make the most of your current resources
Begin by using what you have. Paying for Internet access already? E-mail can be a great way to cut your long-distance telephone costs. It may not be a substitute for your weekly heart-to-hearts with Dad, but it probably should substitute for the "when can we get together again?" calls. Why spend precious money leaving voice mail?

Take the time to get rid of what you don't use. If you're not using it, you won't miss it when it's gone. Donate all unwanted items for a tax deduction, have a garage sale or sell them on eBay. If you have to come up with money for a storage unit for all that stuff, it's time to eliminate that debt.

Pay attention to potential income
Perhaps you have had a hobby for years but have never considered it as a money earner. Take a good look at it now. If you love to scrapbook, consider putting an ad in the paper to teach others how to do the same. At the same time, establish a Web page where others can sign up to learn your craft online.

Could you have old money just waiting to be claimed? Perhaps, you made a move and forgot about an old bank account. There are plenty of free sites that list people who are owed money by insurance companies, banks and utilities. Try MissingMoney and CashUnclaimed.

Ask for a deal
It's that time again when you need to go out and buy a big-ticket item. You know by now to shop around for the best price but are you prepared to ask for a deal. Next time you have your heart set on that ruby ring and you are prepared to drop 3K to make the purchase, stop and think about haggling that price a bit. Don't just assume because you are at a finer jewelry store that the price will be carved in stone. Ask. It never hurts to ask.

Using Good Commonsense and Planning – You Can Survive!!

Armed with the finances that you need to survive, look to the below lists and arm yourself, now, with all of the supplies that you will need in a dire emergency:

Miscellaneous supplies to store up
· 25 pounds laundry soap
· 12 28 oz. bottles dish soap
· 73 rolls toilet paper
· sanitary napkins in sufficient quantity
· 8 gallons bleach (used for sanitation as well as laundry)
· 12 bars hand soap
· 6 24 oz. bottles shampoo
· personal products, such as toothpaste, deodorant
· chainsaw oil and other items to keep things running
· pet foods
· livestock feed
· 55 gallons kerosene for lighting
· 25 gallons Coleman fuel or other lantern fuel

Suggested contents of a good medical kit
A good first aid book
Thermometer

Daily prescription meds for all family
Antibiotics
Ointments for the eye, fungus & cuts
Antidiarhea medication
Pain and anti-inflammatory medication such as aspirin
Burn treatment, such as Burn Free
Iodine/Betadine
Alcohol
Oral electrolytes (for dehydration from fever, diarrhea, stress)
Cold remedies
Cough medicines
Cough drops/throat discs
Bandages
Gauze
Cotton
Surgical tape
Scissors
Hemostats
Tweezers
Needles to remove slivers
A dental kit to patch dentures, replace fillings, etc.)

Checklist for stay-at-home emergencies

- Food and water for family, pets & livestock for at least 14 days; 55 gallons of fresh water will last a family of four for over seven days.
- Daily medications for family for 14 days
- Alternative heat source & fuel
- Alternative cooking source & fuel
- Alternative lighting source & fuel
- Flashlights & batteries
- Transistor, crank or solar radio
- Medical kit
- Matches
- Butane lighters
- Magnesium, flint & steel fire starter

Checklist for vehicle emergency preparedness

Jack & lug wrench
Spare tire
Shovel
Battery jumper cables
Basic tool kit
Fix-A-Flat
Oil

Lighter air pump
Gallon of drinking water
Blankets
Basic first aid kit
Flashlight
Emergency food
Candles with matches
Map
Cell phone or C.B. can
be a life saver

Evacuation Needs
Storage food in large cooler #1

Instant potatoes
Dry milk
Canned tuna
Dehydrated eggs
Dry noodles
Flour
Shortening
TVPs
Dry soup mixes
MREs (military instant Rice
meals; meals ready to eat)
Dry beans
Margarine powder
Dehydrated fruit
Dehydrated vegetables
Tomato powder
Baking powder
Salt
Spices & condiments
Pudding mixes
Cornmeal
Instant coffee, tea, drink mixes
Sugar

Large cooler #2

Frying pan
Large pot
Smaller pot
Mixing bowl, steel (can double as cooking utensil)
Matches & lighters
Toilet paper
Paper towels
Dish towel

Dish soap
Candles
Dish scrubber pad
Bowls for family
Silverware for family
Metal spatula
Roll of duct tape
Small roll of wire
Metal cups for family
Small water filter
Propane stove & tanks
Flashlight & batteries
Hatchet

Sleeping Gear (in large plastic box) Sleeping bags
Candles & lighters
Coleman lantern
Unopened gallon of lantern fuel
Bow saw
Warm socks & jackets
10' x 12' plastic tarp
lightweight tent
Radio

Rifle/shotgun and ammunition (food procurement, signaling, and family protection)

Personal backpacks

Warm clothes
Emergency food
Socks
Stocking hat
Basic fishing gear without rod
Small first aid kit
Space blanket
Flashlight
Roll of wire & rope
Pocket knife
Canteen with cup
Lighter
A few dollars in quarters & bills

IN CASE OF EMERGENCY – BE PREPARED!!

Milton Keynes UK
Ingram Content Group UK Ltd.
UKHW020702040324
438885UK00018B/1194

9 783986 085513